The Skin, Tongue and Nails Speak

Medical Illustrator: Michele Graham
Book Designer: Sue Campbell Graphic Design

ISBN: 978-0-615-60121-2

Published by Unique Perspective Press
Loveland, Colorado
www.donnawild.net

Printed in the United States of America

The Skin, Tongue and Nails Speak:

Observational Signs
of Nutritional Deficiencies

Donna Burka Wild

Contents

CHAPTER THREE: **Fingernails**

Introduction

A CHILD WAKES FROM A TROUBLED SLEEP, AND HIS MOTHER knows something is wrong. Her child normally rises rapidly and is raring to go. Today however, he is listless, missing the sparkle in his eye and the smile on his face. His unwillingness to play or eat is a discerning behavior, unusual for her son. The mother notices his cheeks are flushed and his lips are dry, but his skin is pale and clammy. Increasingly concerned, she asks him to stick out his tongue. It is red, rather than pink, and swollen. She peers into his throat, finding it too is red, inflamed and speckled with little pus sacks. She feels his forehead and takes his temperature. During all this time, she is assessing whether this is something she can handle herself or will she need to call the doctor.

These simple yet caring acts of love and concern, discriminating the difference between wellness and disease, have traditionally been taught to young mothers by their mothers and grandmothers before them. They are observational tools; pearls of healing wisdom passed on to them by the country doctor and local healers.

Throughout history, doctors and healers have used physical observations to monitor the health status of their patients. The preliminary physical examination the medical doctor performs in his office today is a prime example of this. The doctor will take the patient's blood pressure and listen to his heart sounds through a stethoscope to assess the patient's heart health. (*For grammatical consistency, the masculine gender will be used in this book to refer to both doctor and patient.*)

He shines a light into each eye to see if the pupils respond normally by dilating — a remarkably simple test for healthy adrenal function. He then looks through the iris with an opthalmoscope to examine the retina at the back of the eye.

The patient is asked to stick out his tongue. Using a depressor, the doctor moves the tongue aside enabling him to peer into the throat to look at the tonsils to examine their color, looking for signs of inflammation or infection.

The purpose for all this: he is looking for evidence of abnormalities associated with the disease process. This is a standard preliminary exam today, but it is by no means as thorough as it could be.

Historically, before the era of modern medicine, the physician looked at, smelled and even tasted the patient's urine to check for diabetes. In a test for scurvy, a prevalent disease in the days before its cause was clearly know, the physician's assistance would grab hold of the patient's ankles and shake him. While this occurred, the physician would hold an ear cone to the patient's chest, listening for the rattle of bone on bone. The rattle indicated the loss of connective tissue, a sign of advance scurvy. That was long before the use of the sophisticated diagnostic equipment we have today. As primitive as the ancient art of diagnosis was, and despite its serious limitations, it did have some degree of effectiveness.

Unlike the tradition of the past, the physician of today has not been trained to check the tongue's coating and look for abnormalities in its size, shape, color, and for markings and fissures.

By pushing the tongue aside, he misses the opportunity to check for nutritional deficiencies and disease processes that are reflected in changes in the tongue.

There are many such examples of pathological changes that can be detected from straightforward observations by a trained healthcare professional. In addition to the tongue, nutritional deficiencies can be discovered by observing physical changes in the fingernails, eyes, skin and hair.

By researching and studying physical observations of nutritional deficiencies and some simple, non-invasive testing procedures, the practitioner can be aware of an inner lesion or dystrophy (a nutritionally caused abnormality) that may be occurring in the body. This knowledge enables you to be more precise in recommending to your patients nutritional support for the glands, organs and systems involved in their problem. (*Please note: This book uses the definition #2 of a lesion from Stedman's Medical Dictionary: "A pathological change in the tissue"*[1]).

How are the physical observations that can lead to a diagnosis of a potential medical problem defined? They can be defined as overt signs of deviation from the expected norm which can be seen on external portions of the body. Physical observations are simply performed by looking for abnormalities in the skin, hair, eyes, tongue and fingernails of your patients. With proper training, you can correlate those observations with corresponding nutritional deficiencies, which, if left untreated, can lead to dystrophy and a disease process.

---

1 *Stedman's Medical Dictionary*, 27th edition (Baltimore: Lippincott, Williams and Wilkins, 2001), 987.

This book also includes non-invasive tests that can be performed in your office as well as tests that the patient can do at home. With an understanding of the underlying dystrophy, additional laboratory tests can be ordered, if necessary, with which to make the proper diagnosis. These techniques, like other tests, can be up to 77 percent accurate in determining structural or functional changes in tissue[2].

There may be reasons other than nutritional for the lesions identified in this book. *The nutritional suggestions herein are meant to be used in parallel with conventional medical treatment.* It is up to you to ascertain and address underlying causes of the illness. You should also check for all contraindications and drug interactions before making your recommendations.

The purpose of this book is to bring to today's practitioner an awareness of certain bodily signs with the nutritional deficiencies they may indicate and to increase the number of tools you use in that effort.

The Skin, Tongue and Nails Speak intends to teach you to look for nutritional deficiencies that may be involved in the patients' disease processes. You can then recommend to your patients the beneficial dietary food additions, as well as nutritional/herbal supplements that harmoniously support their individual healing processes.

To begin to integrate these ideas into the routine of your physical examinations, start by looking around you. Take a close look at the people with whom you come in contact. Scrutinize

---

2 Broda O. Barnes and Lawrence Galton, *Hypo-Thyroidism: The Unsuspected Illness* (New York: Harper and Row Publishers, 1976), 47.

what is behind the makeup, cosmetic surgeries, injections, nail polish and fake nails that many use to enhance their attractiveness and cover their imperfections. Can you see telltale signs of degeneration and patterns of nutritional deficiencies? They are there, in a significant number of cases.

In this book, you will learn simple, non-invasive and inexpensive ways to recognize and feed nutritional deficiencies that lead to disease pathology. It will enable you to nourish your patients' beauty from the inside, giving to them the gift of true health.

"One of the biggest tragedies of human civilization is the precedents of chemical therapy over nutrition.
It's a substitution of artificial therapy over natural, of poisons over food, in which we are feeding people poisons in trying to correct the reactions of starvation."

— Royal Lee, DDS (1952)

CHAPTER ONE

The Skin

Dark Circles and Swelling Around the Eyes

Dark circles around or under the eyes are often a sign of some deeper disturbance in the body. Afflictions associated with those dark circles may be anemia, fatigue, allergies, nasal congestion, edema, solar radiation damage, parasites, hereditary factors and aging. In this chapter, each of these causations will be addressed individually.

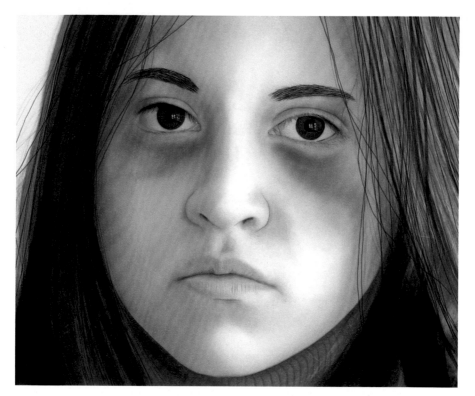

FIGURE 1. Dark circles under the eyes

Anemia Associated with Capillary Fragility

A PROMINENT REASON FOR DARK CIRCLES AROUND THE EYES of a patient may be anemia and poor vascular integrity. They can be caused by the breakdown of hemoglobin in the capillary matrix around eyes. If the walls of the capillaries are weak, they become permeable, and blood will "leak" out of the capillaries into the surrounding tissue and oxidize. This results in a dark pigmentation, like a bruise.

The vitamin P factor, a part of the whole vitamin C complex, supports vascular integrity and prevents capillary fragility[1]. It is the bioflavonoid component of the vitamin C complex, and includes rutin and quercetin, necessary for collagen production. It was named by Albert Szent-Gyorgyi, the Nobel Prize winner for the discovery of vitamin C. He termed it vitamin P for "permeability" because it controls the permeability of the blood vessels. The anti-scorbutic (anti-scurvy) phytochemicals of vitamin P are found in red peppers, buckwheat and citrus, particularly in the rinds of the fruit. They are readily oxidized by air and heat. To get the greatest benefit of those nutrients from fruits and vegetables, it is best to eat the majority of them fresh and raw.

In cases of anemia, it is important to nutritionally support all aspects of hemopoietic (blood cell) production to increase blood quality. Recommend foods or supplements that contain iron, as well as folate, vitamin B12 and the whole vitamin C complex. Consider adding spleen/liver glandulars and bone extracts. Red blood cells are produced in the marrow of the long bones of the

---

1   "Vitamin C as Compared With Synthetic Ascorbic Acid," (Milwaukee, WI: Vitamin Products Company), Form VF-301(R).

body, and in the liver and spleen, therefore the functions of these organs may also need to be nutritionally supported.

Our forefathers ate animal glands and organ meats as well as bone marrow. They understood the organ meat contained more nutrients than the muscle meat. One of the benefits of eating organ meat, especially if it is raw, is that the patient gets all the nutrients in the biologically active form needed for that specific organ. If the patient is opposed to eating organ meat, a glandular supplement in pill form will help with compliance.

Folate is necessary for the creation of red blood cells in the long bones of the body. Foods rich in folate include broccoli, asparagus and liver. Leafy vegetables also supply significant amounts of folate. Spinach, kale, beet greens, endive and Swiss chard are the most common ones your patients will find in their grocery stores.

Vitamin B12 is necessary for the maturation of red blood cells. The best food sources of vitamin B12 are organ meats—liver, kidney and heart—and seafood including sardines, crayfish, trout, herring and raw shellfish, especially oysters and clams. Some naturally occurring B12 is also found in fermented foods such as yogurt, kefir and borsch. Eating fermented foods has the additional benefit of maintaining healthy intestinal flora which, itself, can make small amounts of vitamin B12.

For additional blood-building support, add a fat-soluble chlorophyll supplement. Fat-soluble chlorophyll contains vitamins E, K, F and provitamins A. Chlorophyll, the light absorbing component of green plants, is present in plant sap (or plant "blood") and is similar to the heme molecule in hemoglobin, the oxygen

carrier of human blood. Heme and chlorophyll have similar struc-
tures. At the heart of each molecule is a square, multi-atom complex, at the center of which is bound a metal ion. Chlorophyll
binds a divalent magnesium ion (Mg++), where heme binds a
divalent iron atom (Fe++). Chlorophyll is found abundantly in
green vegetables; it is the molecule that gives them their color.

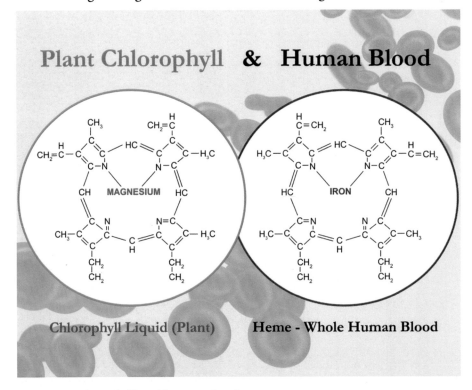

FIGURE 2. Chorophyll and heme molecule

Fat-soluble chlorophyll, containing both vitamin K and
provitamin A, is also useful in supporting other physiological
functions. Recent studies have shown that vitamin K, the prothrombin or clotting factor of blood, along with vitamins A and
B3 (niacinamide), are beneficial to the skin, particularly for dry

skin and pigmentation problems. Dermatologists also have found that vitamin K diminishes the discoloration and puffiness of dark circles under the eyes and bruising on the face. When they combined vitamin K with retinol or vitamin A, there was a significant lightening of the dark circles. The combination also boosts collagen production in the skin[2].

Vitamin B3 has been shown to be an effective skin lightening agent, as well as a natural anti-inflammatory[3]. It is part of the vitamin G complex, a sub-class of the vitamin B complex that is insoluble in alcohol. The vitamin G factors include riboflavin, niacinamide, vitamin B6, folate, biotin, choline and inositol. The properties of the vitamin G complex are nerve-regeneration, nerve-relaxation and vasodilation.

Sluggishness of blood flow under and around the eyes can also contribute to dark circles. Use of the whole vitamin G complex will dilate the capillaries and improve blood flow. This will assist in the removal of the oxidized blood causing the discoloration and puffiness around the eyes.

Fatigue

FATIGUE IS THE NEXT VARIABLE TO CONSIDER WITH REGARD to dark circles. The old wives' tale regarding "beauty sleep" is, in fact, correct. Humans require at least eight hours of sleep every night. Children and teenagers need even more. For patients who have a hard time falling asleep or staying asleep, recommend a calcium supplement before bed. Calcium taken with vitamin F

---

2 "Old Vitamins Learn New Tricks," (*American Academy of Dermatology*, 2005).
3 Ibid.

is especially beneficial for patients who experience charley horse type cramps, as well as restless leg syndrome. Vitamin F is an array of essential fatty acids that works to ionize calcium into the divalent form (Ca++), necessary for transportation from the blood into surrounding tissue. Interestingly, that warm glass of raw, whole milk grandma used to serve before bed, to help with sleep, contained both calcium and vitamin F.

For more difficult sleep cases, it is recommended that the patient take, one hour before bed, a vitamin G supplement, the nerve relaxing fraction of the B vitamin family; and a nerve relaxing trace minerals supplement to calm the body and support the autonomic nervous system. Kelp and alfalfa supplements contain the nerve relaxing, trace minerals calcium, magnesium, iodine and potassium.

An herb that has been traditionally indicated for insomnia is valerian (*Valeriana officinalis*). Valerian is a natural sedative, a relaxing nervine and a hypotensive. It can take up to two weeks for its sleep-inducing abilities to take effect. The use of valerian, as with many herbs, has contraindications. Valerian can potentiate the action of central nervous system depressants such as alcohol, barbiturates and benzodiazepines[4], and may increase sleeping time induced by pentobarbital[5].

Herbal contraindications and drug interactions are why it is logical first choice to heal using nutritional support to correct any underlying deficiencies. There is rarely a food/drug interaction, in

4 *PDR for Herbal Medicines*, Second Edition (Montvale, NJ: Medical Economics Co. Inc., 2000), 784.
5 Sharon Tilgner, *Herbal Medicine from the Heart of the Earth* (Creswell, OR: Wise Acre Press, Inc., 1999), 112.

contrast to the mandating, blocking and depletion of nutrients by pharmaceutical medications.

What if the patient gets plenty of sleep, but still feels and looks fatigued? Look for an underlying problem. Some contributing factors might be exhausted adrenal glands, low functioning thyroid gland, anemia, low-grade infection or insufficient heart function. These will be discussed in detail in later chapters.

Allergies

ALLERGIES TRADITIONALLY HAVE BEEN KNOWN TO CAUSE dark circles under the eyes. Such allergies can be due to air-borne or environmental allergens, or certain foods.

The sinuses and nasal passages are lined with mucous membranes. When an antigen or a particle of a contaminant comes in contact with the mucous membrane, it will irritate the membrane, causing it to produce mucus. This is part of the body's natural defenses intended to keep foreign particles from passing through the mucous membranes into the body.

In an allergy attack, there is a buildup of mucus and histamine, causing an obstruction of flow in the nasal and sinus passages. Nasal congestion, in turn, can cause venous congestion, leading to a pooling of blood under the eyes, resulting in discoloration.

Food allergies can have the same effect. The gastro-intestinal tract is also lined with mucous membranes. An undigested protein from a particle of food can leak though the lining of the intestines into the blood, causing an increase of leukocytes as a defensive cleanup response. Histamines are released and inflammation can occur.

Over consumption of wheat is a common example. Rule this

out by eliminating wheat for a month or so before adding it back into the diet. After being on a restorative nutritional program; the patient may able to consume wheat products a few times per week with little or no detrimental effect. Removing the suspected agent from one's diet for a reasonable time, and then reintroducing it, is a classic diagnostic technique, and is easily undertaken independently by the patient.

Arthur F. Coca, MD, immunologist, researcher and professor, developed a simple test known as the *Coca Pulse Test* to help identify food allergies. (Dr. Coca called it the *Pulse-Dietary Technique.*) It is based on the fact that allergies cause an increase in the pulse rate[6]. This test requires both discipline of the patient and careful supervision of the physician.

Before performing this technique, have the patient remove all suspected food from his diet for a day or two. During that time he needs to take a resting pulse rate for a full 60 seconds several times throughout the day. Quoting Dr. Coca, the resting pulse should be taken at the following times: "Before rising, before retiring, just before each meal, and three times, at 30 minute intervals, after each meal (14 counts each day)"[7].

Record all readings. This determines the patient's normal pulse rate. A healthy person's resting or basal pulse rate should only fluctuate by two beats throughout the day[8]. According to Dr. Coca, greater fluctuations indicate an allergen is being ingested or inhaled.

The *Pulse-Dietary Technique* tests for foods allergens by

---

6   Arthur F. Coca, *The Pulse Test* (New York: Lyle Stuart, 1957), 19.
7   Ibid., 28-30.
8   Ibid., 56.

isolating them in the diet then, testing to see if they cause an acceleration of the pulse. During this test, the patient's meals need to be limited to a single, simple food. On the day the test is started, have the patient take his own pulse before rising, and again before eating breakfast. Thirty minutes after eating a small meal of a suspected allergic food, have the patient take his pulse, and again 60 minutes after the meal.

The patient must keep a diary of the times and the type of foods he ingests along with the pulse rate counts. An increase in the patient's pulse rate of six or more beats after the meal indicates a food allergy. If there is no increase in the pulse rate, there is no allergy and another food can be introduced, repeating the same testing procedure[9].

Inhaled allergens can also be identified with this technique. If you choose to do this work in your practice, obtain Dr. Coca's book, *The Pulse Test*[10], for more detailed information.

Before the allergic patient can be nutritionally supported, it is important that the allergen be removed from the patient's environment. This includes anything the patient is eating, drinking, breathing or coming into contact with, which has been found to cause the allergic reaction. Removing the allergic assault from the body will better enable it to heal.

After the assault is removed, the next step is to restore the health and integrity of the mucous membranes. The nutrients necessary to rebuild healthy mucous membranes are whole vitamins A and C complexes, trace minerals and amino acids.

9 Ibid., 105.
10 Ibid.

The vitamin A complex is found in fish liver oil, kidneys, animal liver, butter and cream. Carrots and leafy green vegetables (beet greens, spinach, kale and broccoli) contain carotene, a pro-vitamin A, which a healthy person can convert into vitamin A. The vitamin C complex is abundant in citrus fruits, berries, cherries, tomatoes, red peppers, raw mushrooms and potatoes. Juicing these fruits and vegetables fresh and raw is an excellent way to optimize the nutrients and make them available in therapeutic portions.

It is wise to check the allergic patient's saliva and urine pH. The body's fluids tend to be alkaline when the body is under allergic assault. Remember, the saliva pH, which reflects that of the blood, should range between 7.0 and 7.2. The urine pH is reflective of the gut and should range between 5.5 and 6.0. Apple cider vinegar is an easily available food to help acidify an alkaline state. Calcium and ammonium chloride salts are available in a supplement form and can be used short term to help lower the body's pH.

For a patient with food allergies, add to his supplements digestive enzymes such as betaine hydrochloride, pepsin, pancreatin, bromelain, lipase, cellulase, papain and amylase. These will help digest his food, removing stress from the digestive tract and allowing it to heal more easily. A probiotic is another important addition to the patient's protocol to help restore healthy flora and the integrity of the gut.

Solar Radiation

EVEN FOR THOSE OF US WHO ARE NOT PROPONENTS OF heavy duty sun blocks, it is important to understand the damage excessive exposure to the sun can do to the skin. Dark circles around the eyes can be one such effect. Building a good base tan is essential for being in the sun for long periods of time. Until then, sun blocks are necessary to prevent damaging burns.

That being said, there is a proper way to tan without causing excess damage to the epithelial tissue. Teach your patients to tan properly by exposing themselves to the sun's rays in short increments. Counsel them to begin tanning by exposing themselves to the sun for only 10 minutes for the first few days, then work up to 20 minutes of exposure time for the next few days, then 30 minutes, and so on. This will allow your patient to tan, without burning and without chemical sun blocks. When the individual had a good base tan, he can stay outside for longer periods of time without the damaging effects of the sun.

Having an adequate supply of calcium and vitamin F and A in the tissue (in this case, the skin) will also help keep the skin from burning and balance the potential effects of hyper-vitaminosis D.

Unprotected skin needs to be exposed to the sun a short time each day for an individual to make the requisite daily amount of vitamin D. When the ultraviolet rays from the sun penetrate the skin, they work with the body's cholesterol to produce vitamin D. A deficiency of vitamin D is now associated with an increase risk of Parkinson's disease[11], multiple sclerosis[12] and cancers of the prostate, breast, ovaries and colon[13].

---

11 Association of Vitamin D Receptor Gene Polymorphism and Parkinson's Disease in Koreans," *J. Korean Med Sci.* 20 (2005), 495-8.
12 "Vitamin D Intake and Incidence of Multiple Sclerosis," *Neurology*, Jan 13, 62 (1), (2004), 60-5.
13 "Vitamin D is associated with a Lower risk of Cancer," *British Medical Journal* (14 Jan) 332:70 (2006), doi:10.1136/bmj.332.7533.70.

Vitamin F is the natural antidote to hyper-vitaminosis D. Vitamin F consists of an array of essential fatty acids —linoleic acid, linolenic acid and arachidonic acid— which have a specific vitamin affect. One of the effects of vitamin F is ionization of calcium to its divalent form (Ca++), making it biologically active and permitting it to be transferred from the blood to the tissues. This action counterbalances the vitamin D effect of increasing blood calcium levels.

Vitamin F is found in a number of foods: unrefined fish liver oil, egg yolks, cream and butter, fish eggs, chlorophyll, raw nuts, avocados, animal fat from pastured animals fed on the fresh, green grass and cold-processed, unrefined, vegetable oils.

Parasites

ANN LOUISE GITTLEMAN, RENOWNED NUTRITIONIST AND author, states that in her clinical experience she has "never seen a person with persistent dark circles who didn't also have an intestinal parasite infestation"[14]. Parasites are associated with conditions such as itchy anus, bruxism, hyperactivity, inability to gain weight, diabetes, bowel disorders and hard-to-eradicate yeast infections.

Because of the life, dormancy and reproductive cycle of parasites, the best parasite lab tests are only 50 percent accurate. This is why the schedule for parasitic eradication is typically 10 days on, then one week off, to allow the eggs to hatch. The program is then resumed: 10 days on and then one week off. This schedule may need to be repeated several times and include family

---

14   Ann Louise Gittleman, with Ann Castro, *The Living Beauty Detox Program*, (San Francisco: Harper, 2000), 128.

members and house pets for complete eradication in difficult cases. Traditionally, the protocol is started three days before the full moon because it has been observed that parasites become more active at that time.

For a safe, non-toxic eradication of intestinal parasites, recommend to your patients the use of proteolytic enzymes. The proteolytic enzymes bromelain, lipase, cellulase, papain, ficin and amylase, taken on an empty stomach, will actually digest the outer protein skeleton of the parasites, resulting in their death.

Garlic has traditionally been used to eradicate parasites. One to two raw cloves eaten each day is a safe amount and can be used in conjunction with the digestive enzymes. Black walnut hulls (*Juglans nigra*) and wormwood (*Artemisia absinthium*) are herbs that also have been used historically for parasitic infection. Be aware of the contraindications associated with both these herbs, and recommend their use appropriately. Whenever working with parasitic or yeast eradication, it is imperative that the patient have two to three good bowel movements each day to prevent the absorption of toxic die-off substances.

Heredity

HEREDITARY OR GENETIC INVOLVEMENT CAN ALSO BE RESPONSIBLE for dark circles. However, there is hope. As Royal Lee, DDS, stated in his 1950 address, "Unfitting the Unborn," to the Academy of Nutrition,

The effects of malnutrition tend to be fixed into the race as hereditary characteristics. You can work them out by feeding the race better, but it takes several generations to get rid of them.

This opinion has been verified by a recent study of epigenetics at Duke University, where, using rats, the researchers determined that a mother's diet can permanently alter the function of her offspring's genes, without altering the DNA sequence. In this study, gene function changed in just one generation, when the mother was fed vitamin and mineral supplements[15].

Aging

WITH THE BIOLOGICAL PROCESSES OF THE AGING, THE FAT pads beneath eyes thin and develop a sunken look. A diet high in fresh fruit and vegetables, fish and healthy fats has been shown to slow that aging process. On the other hand, a diet high in refined carbohydrates, sugars and trans fats, as well as smoking, has been shown to accelerate the aging process, accenting darkness around the eyes.

Edema

PUFFINESS UNDER, ABOVE OR AROUND THE EYES CAN BE DUE to edema. Edema is swelling caused by an excessive accumulation of fluid in or around the tissue. This fluid retention may be caused by inadequate function of the kidneys, thyroid, liver, heart, dietary factors or high blood pressure. The problem for you, the practitioner, now, is to identify and address the underlying cause.

Recommending a natural diuretic such as carbamide from a mineral source will help the body remove the fluid. Carbamide improves the osmotic transfer of fluids through the cell membranes, and it increases the electrical conductivity of the body's natural salts by balancing those electrolytes in all of the body's

---

15   Sandra Blakeslee, "A Pregnant Mother's Diet May Turn the Genes Around," *New York Times*; October 7, 2003. [Quoting from original article in *Molecular and Cellular Biology*, by Dr. Randy Jirtle, August 1, 2003.]

fluids. It functions in this way as a natural diuretic, without depleting potassium from the body.

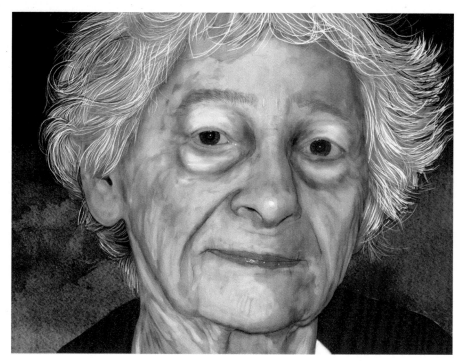

FIGURE 3. Puffiness around the eyes

Dandelion leaf (*Taraxacum officinalis*) and parsley (*Petroselinum crispum*) are herbal diuretics that naturally contain potassium.

Whenever there is edema of the extremities, consider the possibility of a weakened heart. The heart is the backup pump of the body. If the kidneys are not functioning properly the heart is forced to work harder, putting additional stress on the heart muscle and function. It is; therefore, wise to add nutritional support for the heart whenever there is edema in the extremities.

The heart requires protein, a balance of naturally occurring saturated and unsaturated fats, and the whole vitamin complexes B, B4, C, E, E2, F and G, as well as, the minerals calcium, iron, magnesium, potassium and phosphorous. All these nutrients are essential for proper function and the regeneration of healthy heart tissue. It is best to get this sustenance from whole, unadulterated foods or whole food supplements. Eating beef, pork, chicken, or turkey heart is also nutritionally beneficial.

The herb hawthorne leaf (*Crataegus monogyna*) is beneficial for the heart and has no contraindications or side effects. Hawthorne berries (*Crataegus monogyna*) are indicated for support of the vascular system. Beware; however, the two are often mistakenly used interchangeably. It is not uncommon for different parts of the herbal plant to be indicated for different physiological support within the body.

In Chinese medicine, puffiness under the eyes is thought to indicate poor kidney/adrenal function; puffiness above the eyes indicates poor lung function. If the lungs are involved in the puffiness around the eyes, it will be necessary to nutritionally support them as well. The lungs require the whole vitamin A and C complexes, to support the alveoli and the mucous membranes that line the lungs.

In long-term respiratory disorders such as asthma, allergies or pneumonia, there tends to be a disturbance in the histamine-adrenaline metabolism. In such cases, it is important to nutritionally support the adrenal glands for complete resolution. For proper function and synthesis of its hormones, the adrenal glands must have sufficient amounts of the whole vitamin C and G complexes, the tyrosinase enzyme, the amino acid tyrosine (which can be conjugated from tyrosinase) and the minerals copper, sodium and potassium.

Where there is an underlying kidney dysfunction, nutritionally support the kidneys' function and regeneration with whole vitamin A and C complexes. It is beneficial to add to the patient's diet, foods that support the kidneys such as asparagus, black cherries, cranberries, kidney beans and animal kidneys.

CHAPTER TWO

The Tongue

Chinese Tongue Diagnosis

OVERLY SIMPLIFIED, THE THEORY BEHIND CHINESE tongue diagnosis is that the tongue contains an abundance of blood vessels and, therefore, reflects the blood. The tongue is constantly changing by regenerating new tissue. The top-most layer of the tongue's epithelial tissue is fully replaced in two to three days. This is an impressively rapid rate of cell metabolism and growth. Hence, the slightest changes in blood constituents are reflected in the tongue, rapidly altering its color, coating, shape and markings. These tongue changes reflective of blood change, can occur even before symptoms develops within the body.

Below is an illustration of a Chinese tongue map. Utilize it in the physical exam of your patients. Ideally, the patient should have a clean mouth, have recently brushed, and have not had anything to eat or drink in between. Instruct the patient stick out his tongue and tip it down, palette flat. Look for lines, cracks, dents, lumps or abnormalities, and note where they are located. Relate any markings to the corresponding areas of the tongue map.

Many meridians, or energy lines, which correspond to the body's organs, run through the tongue. A tongue map will indicate what areas of the tongue reflect possible dysfunction in the different body organs. It is up to the practitioner to next gather more information regarding the organ and associated conditions. Use the suspect organ as focal point of the observational exam.

Ask the patient pertinent, symptomatic questions regarding disorders of the concerned organ, and order diagnostic tests, if necessary, for further information.

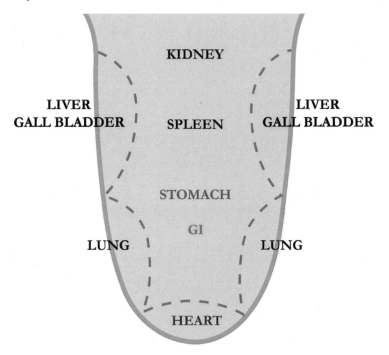

FIGURE 4. Tongue map

The Healthy Tongue

WHAT SHOULD A HEALTHY TONGUE LOOK LIKE? THE tongue's normal color should be light red or pink. The tongue should also be slightly wet with a thin, white coating. Its shape should be thin, not swollen, without markings, wrinkles, fissures, bumps or teeth marks. If you see any of these on your patient's tongue, refer to the tongue map to identify which organs these lesions may be reflecting.

The tongue should also be flexible, supple and mobile. Make

sure the patient is able to move his tongue in and out of the mouth and side to side. According to Chinese medicine, the tongue's mobility reflects that of the mind. In other words, the greater the range of motion and flexibility of the patient's tongue, the more acute his sharpness of mind and the degree of his coordination.

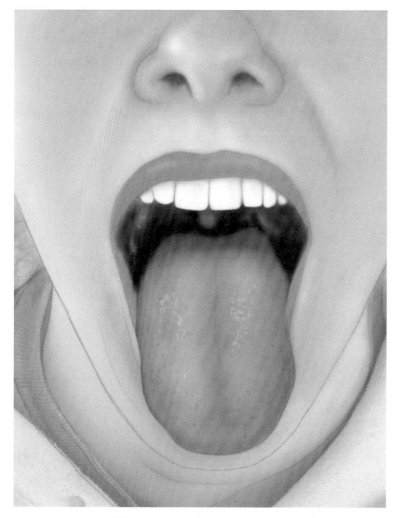

FIGURE 5. *The healthy tongue*

The Tongue as an Indicator of Nutrient Deficiencies

ALTHOUGH CHINESE TONGUE DIAGNOSIS IS INCLUDED IN this chapter, the nutritional deficiencies that are indicated in the tongue are referenced from the vast library of published medical and nutritional text books. This book is meant only to cover underlying nutritional deficiencies which may contribute to the presence of the lesions mentioned and discussed. The practitioner must also consider other idiopathic and pharmacological involvements.

Due to its rapid cellular metabolism rate, nutritional deficiencies are quickly reflected in the tongue. For example, as malnutrition progresses so will atrophy of the taste buds. The scientifically proven, nutritional deficiencies related to tongue changes discussed in this chapter are valuable in any nutritional assessment.

The appendix includes a chart to help utilize the information in this chapter while performing a tongue exam on your patients.

Riboflavin Deficiency

IN A RIBOFLAVIN (VITAMIN B2) DEFICIENCY, THE TONGUE takes on a purplish or magenta color[1]. In Chinese medicine, this is also an indication of blood stasis. Be alert for associated circulation problems. Interestingly, riboflavin has a vasodiolating effect. In conjunction with its lipotrophic properties of breaking up fat deposits, it increases circulation. Besides a color change of the tongue, a vitamin B2 deficiency may show itself as angular

---

1   Michael Zimmermann, *Micronutrients in Health and Disease* (New York: Thieme Publishing, 2001), 13.

stomatitis and/or inflamed buccal mucosa[2]. It is not uncommon to be accompanied by a sore throat. Atrophy of the taste buds is another symptom of a vitamin B2 deficiency[3].

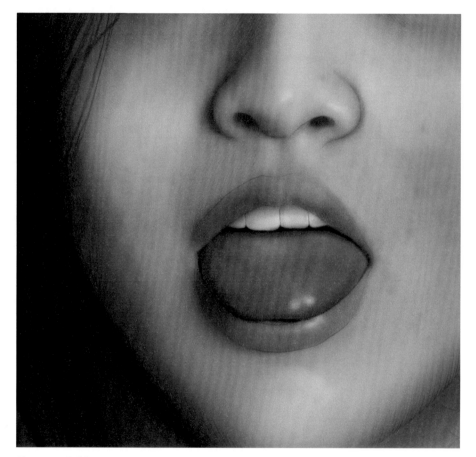

FIGURE 6. Magenta tongue

Riboflavin is protein-bound in foods and often occurs with other B vitamins. Rich food sources include nutritional yeast,

2   H.K. Biesalski, and P. Grimm, *Pocket Atlas of Nutrition* (Stuttgart: Thieme Publishing, 2004), 174.
3   Michael Zimmermann, *Micronutrients in Health and Disease* (New York: Thieme Publishing, 2001), 13.

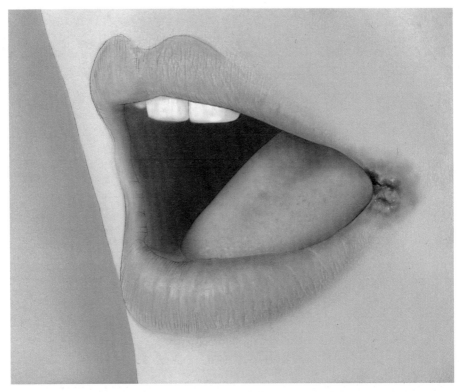

Figure 7. Angular stomatitis

sprouted grains (particularly those of unrefined bran and germ), liver, brain, mushrooms and dairy, especially raw cheeses and yogurt.

Therapeutically, support the underlying deficiency in your patients with a food-based, vitamin G supplement to ensure that the riboflavin is balanced with it co-factors.

Niacinamide Deficiency

GLOSSITIS IS ONE SIGN OF A NIACINAMIDE OR VITAMIN B3 deficiency and is extremely uncomfortable for the patient. Swelling and redness start at the tip and lateral margins of the tongue and progresses to cover the entire surface. As the deficiency advances, ulcers on the tongue may develop[4].

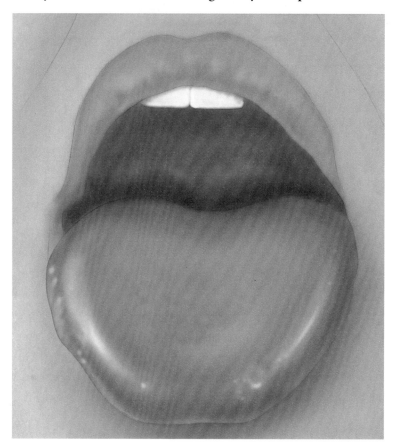

FIGURE 8. Glossitis

Besides the painful and inflamed tongue, there may also be fissures on the lips[5]. In a vitamin B2 deficiency, the fissures are at

4   Robert P. McCombs, *Internal Medicine in Clinical Practice* (Philadelphia: W.B. Saunders Co, 1943), 209.
5   Michael Zimmermann, Burgerstein's *Handbook of Nutrition: Micronutrients in the Prevention and Therapy of Disease* (Stuttgart: Thieme Publishing, 2001), 40.

the corners of the mouth; with a vitamin B3 deficiency, the cracks are actually on the lips themselves.

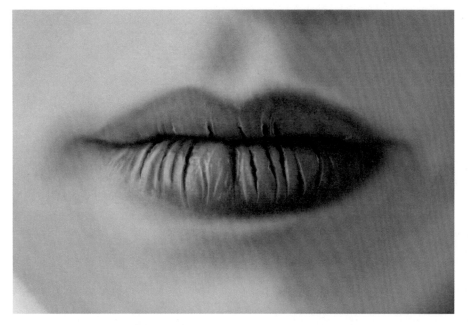

FIGURE 9. Fissures on lips

Niacinamide, nicotinic acid and vitamin B3 are one and the same nutrient. Niacin is the synthetic form. Niacinamide is required for energy production, health of the skin, mucus membranes, digestive and nervous systems, DNA reproduction and repair, as well as fat and cholesterol metabolism. Niacinamide is found in liver, lean meats, poultry, peanuts and fish (especially tuna and halibut).

Niacinamide works synergistically with vitamin B6, B2 and tryptophan. Ideally, the patient should be encouraged to make dietary changes that include rich food sources of these nutrients. This synergistic combination naturally occurs in many of the foods we eat, with the exception of corn. Corn contains a nicotinic acid inhibitor that can be deactivated by soaking the corn in lime or alkali.

Whole food supplements allow the practitioner to give a therapeutic dose of a nutrient in combination with its synergist co-factors in a pill form the patient is normally used to taking.

Therapeutically, recommend a whole vitamin G complex supplement. Vitamin G is part of the B vitamin complex and is comprised of vitamin B2, B3, B6, choline, inositol, folate and biotin. (These components tend to be insoluble in alcohol.) The vitamin G complex has properties of vasodilation, nerve relaxation and nerve regeneration.

Vitamin G was named after Dr. Joseph Goldberger, MD, who was a U.S. military doctor at the beginning of the twentieth century. He discovered the need for these combined nutrients in his search for a cure for, and prevention of, pellagra. The word pellagra comes from the Italian, *pelle agra*, meaning rough skin. This disease devastated Italy and other parts of Europe in the 1700s, and in the early 1900s was a bane to the poor population in the southern United States.

Pellagra is thought of as a nutritional deficiency disease of the past, but it is still present in our population today. When you look at the tongue, lips and skin of your patients, you may see signs of preclinical pellagra. This is especially true of patients with gastrointestinal problems where there is poor digestion and nutrient absorption, or in alcoholics who prefer to get their calories from alcohol, not from food, leading inevitably to malnourishment.

Early Warning Signs of Pellagra

It is important to recognize the signs and symptoms of pellagra. Advancing beyond the inflamed tongue and cracked lips, mild cases of pellagra include neurasthenia, dyspepsia and eczema. Gone unrecognized, these preclinical symptoms will gradually increase in intensity. The patient will suffer from loss of weight, strength and appetite, insomnia, vertigo, headaches, irritability, loss of memory, depression and constipation (which will progress into diarrhea if left untreated). Other symptoms include abdominal pain, alimentary problems, heart palpitation, nervousness, inability to concentrate and pain in the limbs[6].

As the disease progresses, more obvious clinical signs appear. Dermatitis develops in the form of a red rash, eczema or as areas of a shiny, highly pigmented thickening of the skin, sometimes occurring with cracks.

Casal's necklace is a well-known pellagra rash that is identified by a beaded rash or lesions that wraps around the neck line. The rash is named after Gaspar Casal, a physician of Oviedo, Spain, who studied pellagra extensively during its European outbreak in the 1700s. In a "reverse" Casal's, the red, beaded eruptions appear on the back of the neck. Another form of dermatitis is the butterfly rash of pellagra, where a red rash develops on the cheeks and nose resembling the shape of a butterfly.

As pellagra progresses, the early complaint of constipation transitions to diarrhea, and the nervousness and depression progress into dementia. The sclera of the eyes turns a bluish color, and

---

6   F. Bicknell and F. Prescott, *The Vitamins in Medicine* (New York: Grune & Stratton, 1958,) 354 - 356.

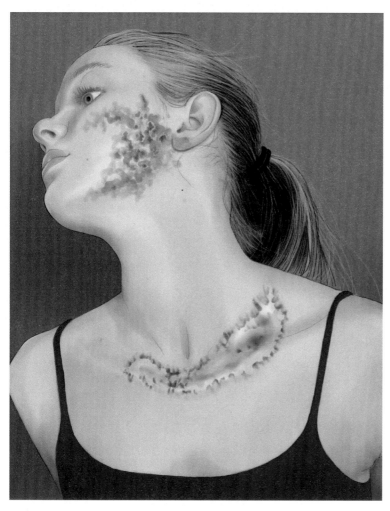

FIGURE 10. Casal's necklace with butterfly rash

the patient will develop a dull lifeless stare[7]. Pellagra is known for its three Ds: Dermatitis, Diarrhea and Dementia. Left untreated, a fourth D can occur — **Death!**

In most cases the underling nutritional deficiencies related to pellagra will resolve themselves in six to nine months if the

---

7   Ibid., 356.

patient adopts a nutritious diet consisting of liver, organ meats, red meat, nutritional yeast, black strap molasses, raw dairy products, egg yolks and green leafy vegetables.

Therapeutically, with the patient's dietary changes include a whole-food based, vitamin G complex supplement to ensure compliance.

Iron Deficiency

A VERY PALE, LIGHT COLORED TONGUE IS ASSOCIATED WITH anemia caused by an iron deficiency. The tongue has lost its

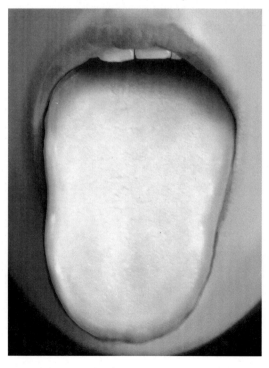

healthy pink color and has paled. With an iron deficiency, it is not uncommon for the tongue to be sore, accompanied with atrophy of the taste buds and/or by angular stomatitis.

Poor circulation in the body may be another reason for the loss of the tongue's natural color. For information on circulatory support, refer to Chapter Three under *Lack of Lunulas*.

Patients with iron deficien-

FIGURE 11. Pale tongue

cy anemia may display a pale complexion and/or dark circles around their eyes. They will typically fatigue and chill easily, especially in the extremities. Other symptoms include brittle and spooning nails, heart palpitations, rapid heart rate, and rapid breathing upon exertion[8]. These symptoms indicate the body is actually compensating for symptoms of suffocation!

The lack of oxygen resulting from the iron deficiency is caused by a reduced size of the red blood cells coupled with a reduction in its hemoglobin content. Hemoglobin and the vitamin C complex carry oxygen in the blood[9].

An interesting side note is the fact that the E2 factor of the whole vitamin E complex acts as an oxygen conserving factor in the body[10].

Another observational test indicating a possible anemia is the "nail press." Notice the color of the patient's unpolished nails. They should be light pink in color. Press down on one of the nail beds. The nail should lose it light pink color and become white. Upon release of pressure, the nail should return to its pink color within three seconds. Taking longer for color to return to the nail bed may denote an anemic condition.

Use caution when recommending ferrous sulfate for anemia. It is irritating to the stomach's mucosa and can cause bowel changes. Rather, choose a food source or whole supplement to overcome nutritional deficiencies. The best bioavailable food sources of iron include red meat, liver and organ meats, fish, oysters and poultry. These food sources contain heme iron which is

---

8 Jane Higdon, *An Evidence Base Approach to Vitamins and Nutrition* (New York: Thieme Publishing, 2003), 139.

9 "Cataplex C" (Milwaukee, WI: Vitamin Product Company, 1934), and Judith A. De Cava, *The Real Truth About Vitamins and Antioxidants* (Columbus, OH: Brentwood Academic Press, 1996), 183.

10 "Vitamin E2," *Index of Product Bulletins* (Milwaukee,WI: Vitamin Product Company, circa 1940's).

more readily absorbed than iron from non-heme sources[11] . Less bioavailable food sources of iron—iron in the non-heme form—include spinach and dark leafy green vegetables, egg yolks and black strap molasses.

Therapeutically, recommend the use of an iron supplement from a liver source, which it contains folate and vitamin B12. Folate stimulates red blood cell production in the long bones of the body; vitamin B12 is necessary to stimulate the maturation of red blood cells[12]. Ideally, the iron supplement should be balanced with zinc and copper, respective to their proper blood ratios.

If the food-based supplement is derived from liver, those minerals will be naturally occurring. Isolated minerals and vitamins can be used therapeutically for short term healing in the body. However, for long term healing, it is important to respect the natural balance of nutrients in the body. An abundance of one nutrient can accentuate a deficiency of other nutrients.

Cobalamin (Vitamin B12) Deficiency

A RED AND INFLAMED TONGUE IS REFERRED TO AS "BEEFY" in Chinese medicine. A red and inflamed tongue may indicate a cobalamin or vitamin B12 deficiency. With this deficiency, the tongue is usually very sore and can lose its coating, giving it a glossy appearance[13].

Vitamin B12 is critical for the maturation of red blood cells.

11   Jane Higdon, *An Evidence Base Approach to Vitamins and Nutrition* (New York: Thieme Publishing, 2003), 141.

12   Arthur C. Guyton, *Text Book of Medical Physiology* (Philadelphia: W.B. Saunders Co, 1986), 45.

13   Lynn S. Bickley, and Peter G. Szilagyi, *Bates' Guide to Physical Examination and History Taking*, 8th ed. (Philadelphia: Lippincott Williams & Wilkins, 2003), 206.

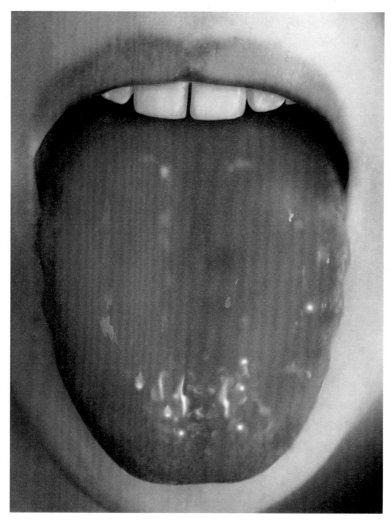

FIGURE 12. Red, inflamed tongue

The failure of red blood cells to mature is known as pernicious anemia, a vitamin B12 deficiency disease. Other symptoms of vitamin B12 deficiencies are weakness and fatigue, irritability, hostility, forgetfulness, confusion, poor memory, agitation, psychosis, depression, numbness and tingling of the extremities, unstable gait, inability to convert homocysteine to methionine and impaired cell reproduction[14].

Vitamin B12 is found in meats, especially organ meats, as well as in fish, mussels, dairy products and eggs. Fermented foods such as sauerkraut, tempeh, yogurt, kefir, borscht, kimchi and beer have trace amounts of vitamin B12. Eating fermented foods also promote healthy intestinal flora from which the body can make vitamin B12.

Vitamin B12 assimilation is diminished by the use of antacids and hydrochloric acid blocking agents. A substance known as "the intrinsic factor" is necessary for the absorption of B12 from the gut. The intrinsic factor and hydrochloric acid are both secreted by the parietal cells in the gastric mucosa[15]. Because they are secreted by the same cells, drugs which block the production and release of hydrochloric acid, unfortunately, will have the same effect on the intrinsic factor. This is compounded by the fact that stomach acids are necessary for the release of vitamin B12 from the protein to which it is bound in foods[16], contributing to or causing, a vitamin B12 deficiency.

Therapeutically, recommend a vitamin B12 supplement that contains the intrinsic necessary for B12 absorption in the ileum.

In Chinese medicine, this "beefy tongue" is considered a chi deficiency. Chi is a term used for the body's vital life force energy. The herb traditionally prescribed to increase chi is

14   Michael Zimmermann, *Micronutrients in Health and Disease* (New York: Thieme Publishing, 2001), 25.
15   Arthur C. Guyton, *Text Book of Medical Physiology* (Philadelphia: W.B. Saunders Co, 1986), 75.
16   Jane Higdon, *An Evidence Base approach to Vitamins and Nutrition* (New York: Thieme Publishing, 2003), 57.

Astragalus membranaceus. It is used in combination with other herbs that specifically direct the body's energy and its circulation. Astragalus has immune enhancing, adaptogenic and cardio-tonic properties. Due to its warming properties, the administration of Astragalus should be discontinued during a fever or acute infection. Remember when using herbs to check for contraindications and drug interactions.

Fissures and Cracks Covering the Tongue

CRACKS AND FISSURES COVERING THE TONGUE CAN BE A sign of an advanced B-vitamin deficiency. Psychological symptoms such as depression, dementia, psychosis and neurosis are

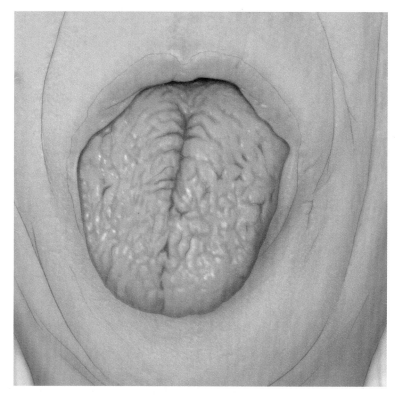

FIGURE 13. *Fissured and cracked tongue*

typically seen in these patients. It is essential for the patient to eat a balanced diet of meat, fish, poultry, dairy, nutritional yeast, brown rice and unprocessed grains. This will ensure getting the complete array of B and G components of the vitamin B complex necessary to correct the underlying deficiency.

Where the deficiency is advanced, therapeutically recommend a whole food vitamin B and vitamin G complex supplement, nutritional yeast and a vitamin B12 supplement that contains the intrinsic factor.

In Chinese tongue diagnosis terminology, this is a chi and yin deficiency. Chi is the body's energy or life force; blood is yin. Interestingly, B vitamins are necessary for energy production and for the hemopoietic system.

Other Telltale Signs of the Tongue

Thick Tongue

A THICK TONGUE IN A CHILD IS A SIGN OF CONGENITAL HY-
pothyroidism. The tongue does not fit in the space provided
for it. In adults, a thick tongue may either be an indication of
hypothyroidism or a sign of a pituitary deficiency. In the 1960s,
medical examiners performed studies on the varying symptoms of
hypothyroidism. In these studies, 60 to 80 percent of their patients had thick tongues [17].

Using observational signs, it is possible to determine whether the patient has a thyroid insufficiency versus a pituitary insufficiency.

In hypothyroidism the body's metabolic and oxidative rate is decreased due to the inadequate production or release of thyroid hormones. The body's energy and temperature run low. Due to this, a patient who has a low functioning thyroid

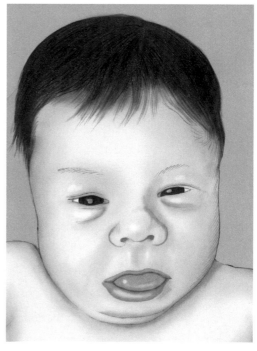

FIGURE 14. *Thick tongue associated with congenital hypothyroidism*

17 Broda O. Barnes and Lawrence Galton, *Hypo-Thyroidism: The Unsuspected Illness* (New York: Harper and Row Publishers, 1976), 23.

typically feels cold. He could have cold extremities and feel chilled down to the very core of his body even when others feel comfortable. He is cold because his body temperature runs below normal.

The thyroid gland is the body's metabolic regulator. One of its functions is to maintain a constant body temperature of 97.8 to 98.6 degrees Fahrenheit. This is optimal for the body's temperature sensitive processes to occur. These temperature sensitive processes include many of the chemical reactions involved in the utilization of the vitamins, minerals and enzymes. If the body's temperature is compromised, either higher or lower, so are many of its functions.

Broda O. Barnes, MD, a physiologist, medical doctor and professor of endocrinology, researched thyroid function and related diseases in the 1950s and 60s. He believed the body's basal (or resting) temperature, was a reliable reflection of an individual's thyroid hormone function inside the cell, where it controls the rate of oxidation (or burning) of foodstuff for fuel. Through testing thousands of individuals, he determined the optimal basal temperature (taken orally or axillary) should be 97.8 to 98.2 degrees Fahrenheit. He observed his hypothyroid patients' basal temperatures ran below 97.8 degrees and his hyperthyroid patients' ran basal temperatures above 98.2 degrees[18].

As Dr. Barnes pointed out, there are conditions other than thyroid disease which may produce an abnormal temperature reading. An infection or ovulation will cause a temporary elevation in the body's temperature. Starvation, or a pituitary or

18   Ibid, 46.

adrenal gland insufficiency, can also produce a lower temperature. To which he writes, "But starvation is certainly not difficult to rule out—and some thyroid is frequently indicated, anyhow, for the other conditions.... Although the basal temperature test is not 100 percent specific for thyroid function, the simple procedure is remarkably successful in uncovering hypothyroidism"[19].

To conduct the *Barnes' Basal Temperature Test for Thyroid Function* use of a mercury or fertility thermometer that takes a ten minute read is best. Purchase a supply to keep in your office to loan or sell to your patients. (You can still buy these from fertility clinics and the internet. Also check with your medical supplier.) Or, have your patient ask their mother, grandmothers or aunts if they still have a mercury thermometer in their medicine cabinet.

To perform the test:

BEFORE RETIRING FOR THE NIGHT, PLACE A MERCURY THERmometer (shaken down well), a pad of paper and a pen on the bed stand. First thing upon waking, hold the thermometer snugly in the arm pit against the skin (axillary) for ten minutes. Record the reading then rise and start the day.

Have the patient do this test for three to five days and then average the temperatures. Again, the optimal temperature should be 97.8 to 98.2 degrees Fahrenheit. A degree lower is indicative of hypothyroidism; a degree higher indicative of hyperthyroidism[20].

Basal means resting, so the temperature must be taken immediately upon waking. Not after writing in a journal, contemplating the day ahead or getting up to urinate. In compensation for

---

19 Ibid, 47.
20 Ibid, 46.

their lower body temperature; hypothyroid people tend to hold fluids around their middle to keep the body's core warm. Getting out of bed to urinate will change the reading of the test.

For a menstruating female this test should be performed during days one to fourteen of her cycle; day one being the day the bleeding begins. A woman's body temperature changes with the onset of ovulation. When a woman ovulates, her basal temperature will rise 0.4 to 0.8 degrees. The basal temperature remains slightly elevated until the menses starts again[21]. Planned Parenthood uses this basal temperature test as part of their fertility awareness programs with healthy couples having difficulties conceiving and as a contraceptive method.

The low thyroid patient is disposed to gain weight easily or to be overweight. The increased weight, however, tends to be distributed around the waist or mid-torso, causing an enlarged waist and abdomen, with a full trunk or barrel shaped. There is a difference of less than ten inches in his waist/hip measurement[22]. This is in part due to his body retaining fluids through the middle section, trying to keep the core of his body warm. He may also have puffy skin (myxedema) and a thick neck (caused by a goiter). The patient may complain of thin hair, dry skin or brittle nails.

Signs of hypothyroidism include:

- **Thick, flat tongue**
- **Malaise**
- **Dry, coarse skin**

---

21   "Ways to Chart Your Fertility Pattern", Planned Parenthood of the Rocky Mountains; plannedparenthood.org.
22   Louis L. Rubel, MD, *The GP and the Endocrine Glands* (Decatur IL, 1959), 81.

- Lethargy
- Slow speech
- Sensitive to cold
- Constipation
- Edematous eyelids
- Frequent winking and blinking
- Decreased perspiration
- Brittle nails and hair
- Alopecia
- Weight gain
- Edema
- Anemia
- Hoarseness of voice
- Clotty menstrual bleeds
- Dysmenorrhea and/or menorrhalgia
- Depression
- Bradycardia
- Digestive disorder
- Thin outer 1/3 of eyebrows
- High cholesterol
- Hypoglycemia
- Goiter
- Lack of libido
- Infertility and miscarriages
- Cretinism/Down syndrome (associated with iodine deficient hypothyroidism)

The thyroid requires vitamins A, B, C, D, E and F complexes (essential fatty acids); the amino acid tyrosine; and the trace minerals iodine, iron, selenium, magnesium and zinc to produce and utilize its hormones. The amino acid tyrosine is bound to iodine in the thyroid to create thyroid hormones. Three iodine

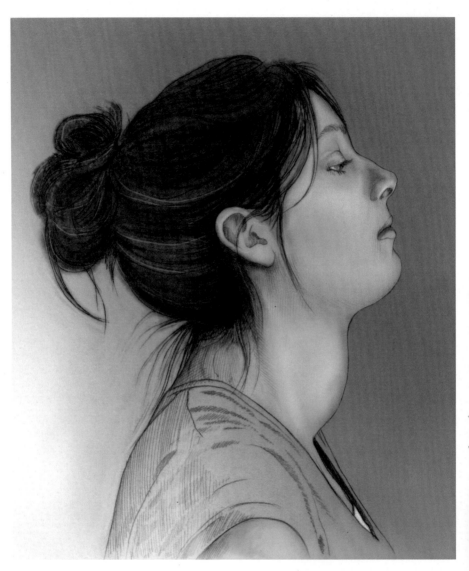

FIGURE 16. Goiter

molecules are bound to tyrosine to create T3; four iodine molecules are bound to tyrosine to create T4. Foods high in iodine
include kelp and other sea vegetables, fish liver oils, shellfish and
ocean fish.

Lugol's solution, a pharmaceutical preparation of iodine and potassium iodide, has been used since the late 1800s for thyroid disorders. It is now available in pill form. A protein-bound iodine/iodide, food-based supplement is preferable. An adjunctive recommendation can be kelp tablets. Kelp is high in iodine plus other trace minerals from the sea.

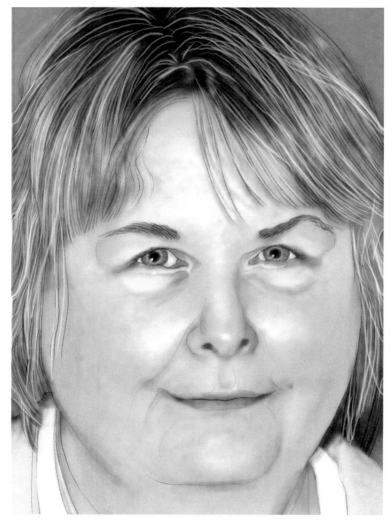

FIGURE 15. Myxedema

Patients with insufficient pituitary function are typically indecisive and cry easily. They frequently take a long time to make up their minds or they keep changing their minds. They cry watching sentimental TV commercials or when listening to a sad song on the radio. A pear shape is the typical body type of a pituitary challenged person. Their bodies are slender on top with disproportionately large hips and thighs. When they gain weight, it tends to be carried low. The term "pituitary apron" refers to that flabby, fatty, flesh of the abdomen that hangs down over the pelvic area.

It is important to remember that the pituitary gland is the master endocrine organ. It regulates the thyroid, adrenal glands, pancreas and gonads. To be able to produce hormones, the pituitary requires the whole vitamin E complex, the trace mineral manganese and B vitamins.

If you are at all uncertain of the thick tongue's origin, order a complete blood panel, including TSH, T3 and T4 values. Remember, T3 is primarily the active form of the thyroid hormone thyroxin, and T4 is primarily the storage form. TSH, the thyroid-stimulating hormone, is produced in the pituitary and therefore also reflects the pituitary's involvement.

Migratory Glossitis or "Geographic Tongue"

IN MIGRATORY GLOSSITIS, OR GEOGRAPHIC TONGUE, THE tongue has a patchy white coating on it. The patches actually resemble land masses of a map. This condition may indicate a yeast infection. Left untreated, it can potentially develop into thrush and become systemic.

Other symptoms and conditions relating to yeast and fungal

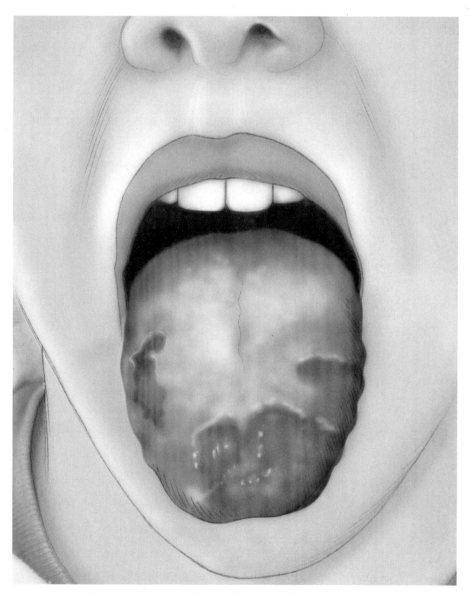

FIGURE 17. Migratory glossitis—"geographic tongue"
infections include rashes, itching, gas, flatulence, abdominal
bloating, vaginal discharge, jock itch, athlete's foot, cradle cap
and dandruff.

If you suspect your patient has a yeast infection have them perform the *Candida Sputum Test*. It is a simple test for systemic fungal infections in the body that can be conducted in your office or in the patient's home.

This test is best performed first thing upon rising in the morning, before the patient puts anything into their mouth. That means before the patient brushes his teeth, drinks his morning cup of coffee, juice or water. Albeit, this test can still be indicative if performed at another time in your office.

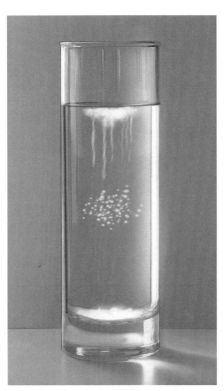

Instruct the patient spit into a clear glass filled with water. Have the patient observe the sputum in the glass of water, every 15 minutes, for the one hour.

If the patient observes strings (like legs) traveling down into the water from the saliva floating on the top, cloudy saliva that sinks to the bottom of the glass, or cloudy specks suspended in the water, then the saliva is carrying a fungus, indicating a possible fungal overgrowth in the body. If there are no strings and the saliva is still floating after one hour, the patients can be considered free of Candida and other fungal overgrowth.

FIGURE 18. Candida sputum test

There is flora on our skin, in our mouths, intestinal tract and vaginal tract of women. Many types of yeast (Candida being one of them) and bacteria live in a natural balance in the flora. Candida in the intestines acts like a garbage collector. It actually engulfs decomposing food, tissue and other debris[23]. A reduction of the normal bacteria in the flora can cause the Candida to proliferate and overgrowth occurs. A healthy immune system will keep Candida growth in check. When the immune system becomes compromised, Candida can grow excessively and spread to places it does not belong.

The first choice in nutritionally supporting a patient suffering from a yeast or fungal infection should be the use of acidophilus or mycelium yeast. These healthy yeast products change any sugar or carbohydrate in the diet to lactic acid. Lactic acid changes the pH in the large intestines and bowel to its natural acidic state, an environment in which healthy, beneficial flora can proliferate and thrive, starving out the Candida infection.

Recommend the patient add to his diet lacto-fermented vegetables such as sauerkraut, kimchi, pickles and kvas. Please note there may be bowel discomfort, gas, belching, cramping and flatulence for a couple of weeks while the flora is re-establishing itself.

A quality yogurt can also be used to help re-establish healthy flora. The acidophilus bacteria in yogurt and kefir will primarily convert lactose, or milk sugar, into lactic acid. If you choose to use an acidophilus and bifidus bacteria supplement, recommend the patient ingest dairy products along with it, to get the greatest benefit.

For geographic tongue and thrush, it is preferable to have the

---

23 Judith DeCava, CNC, LNC, "The Yeast Connection", *Nutrition News and View*, Vol.8, No 1; Jan/Feb 2004.

patient chew acidophilus or mycelium yeast wafers. This will give the additional benefit of working topically, as well as systemically, to change the flora pH and encourage the growth of healthy flora in both the mouth and the intestines. Add garlic to the patient's protocol, either as fresh, raw cloves, or in a supplement form. Garlic's anti-fungal components will cross the blood barrier and help combat a systemic yeast infection. The herbs pau d' arco (*Tabebuia impetiginosa*) and cat's claw (*Uncaria tomentosa*) have antifungal properties, as well, and may be added to the protocol. Remember, when using herbs, to check for contraindications and drug-herbal interactions.

The patient should be having two to three bowel movements per day when on a flora rebuilding protocol. The toxins that result from the die-off of the yeast cells can cause uncomfortable symptoms in the patient. Take the patients off all sugars, refined carbohydrates, chlorinated and brominated water (whether it's drinking, bathing or swimming); these can cause and perpetuate a yeast infection.

With geographic tongue or thrush, have your patient replace the toothbrush he is using with a new one. Brushing their teeth with a toothbrush that is infected with yeast spores will continue to re-infecting the patient. It is important that these patients change their toothbrush on a regular basis.

Do not overlook that yeast infections can be sexually transmitted. In the case of yeast or fungal infections, it is necessary to treat both partners in the relationship. Only the treatment of both partners will simultaneously eliminate the chance of re-infection.

White, Coated, "Hairy" Tongue

WHITE COATING, OR A "HAIRY" TONGUE, AS IT IS ALSO RE-
ferred to, looks as if there is a fuzzy debris growing on the tongue.
This is indicative of sluggish digestion.

In Chinese tongue diagnosis, it means there is too much heat
in the body. Traditionally, the recommendation is to do a "cleansing of the heat"— a cooling, digestive cleanse. Digestive enzymes
alone will not resolve this condition. They do, however, enhance
digestion and are a recommended adjunct to an intestinal detoxification protocol. Intestinal cleanses include elimination of most
foods, especially refined and packaged foods, and replacing them
with low-glycemic fruits and certain vegetables and herbs.

It is important to restrict caloric intake while undertaking
a cleanse. This will allow the body to eliminate toxins stored in
the body, as opposed to the elimination of toxins which are introduced or produced by eating daily meals. The purpose of the
regimen is to stimulate Phase I and Phase II liver detoxification,
to clean and heal the intestinal tract and restore healthy intestinal
flora, all of which are intended to ensure maximum assimilation
of nutrients.

Methyl donor foods stimulate Phase I and Phase II liver detoxification. For a cooling cleanse they include red peppers, garlic,
beets, beet tops, spinach, mushrooms, radishes, asparagus, oranges, seafood, brewer's yeast, eggs and cruciferous vegetables including cabbage, broccoli, Brussels sprouts, cauliflower and kale[24].

Cleanses should be done with discretion. Detoxifying the

---

24   Craig Cooney, and Bill Lawren, *Methyl Magic* (Kansas City: Andrews
McMeel Publishing, 1999), 48-57.

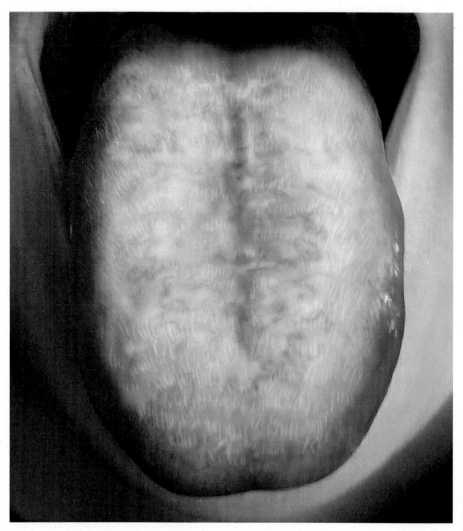

FIGURE 19. White, coated, "hairy" tongue

liver will eliminate drugs more quickly from the body. If the patient is reliant on a pharmaceutical drug for survival (such as a
heart medication or anti-seizure drugs), then a liver detoxification
would be contraindicated. Warning: *never* detoxify a pregnant or
lactating woman! The toxins can cross through the membranes

of the placenta, affecting the fetus; as well as accumulating in breast milk.

Atrophic Glossitis

ATROPHIC GLOSSITIS, OR A SMOOTH TONGUE, OCCURS when the tongue loses its healthy coating. The taste buds will eventually atrophy and the tongue is often sore. This condition usually indicates a B vitamin deficiency, specifically, that of riboflavin, niacinamide, pyridoxine, vitamin B12 or folate. The tongue may also exhibit these changes in the case of an iron deficiency. Interestingly, a riboflavin deficiency affects iron metabolism[25].

With atrophic glossitis, your skills as a practitioner will be especially valuable in determining which specific deficiency may be contributing to the tongue changes.

Therapeutically, recommend to the patient a whole food vitamin B and vitamin G supplement along with a nutritional yeast product, to ensure he is getting the full spectrum of the vitamin B complex. Prescribe a food-based iron supplement if you believe the atrophic glossitis is cause by an iron deficiency.

Determining a nutritional deficiency in a patient is like piecing together a puzzle. It is essential to know the signs and symptoms of nutritional deficiencies. The practitioner must also understand which nutrients the specific organ, gland or system needs in order to function and regenerate properly. A firm knowledge of these two elements will greatly simplify the task of creating a nutritional protocol.

Part of your job as the practitioner is to recognize the physical

---

25   H.K. Biesalski and P. Grimm, *Pocket Atlas of Nutrition* (Stuttgart: Theime Publishing, 2004), 174.

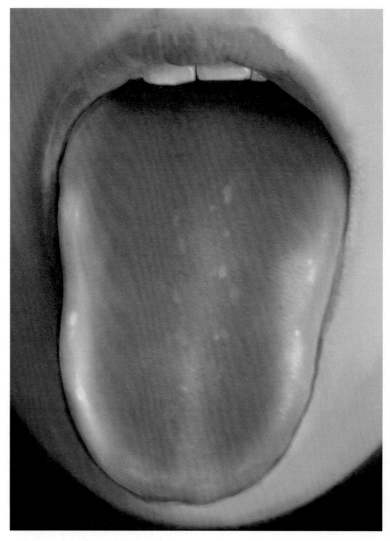

FIGURE 20. Atrophic glossitis

symptoms of dystrophy and ask the right questions to determine the precise deficiencies. This will also help to determine which specific lab work and/or test to order, minimizing both cost and stress for the patient.

Using atrophic glossitis as an example, some signs to look for in a patient, as well as some questions to ask to help determine specific nutritional deficiencies, are noted below.

In a *riboflavin (vitamin B2) deficiency*, look closely at the tongue and lips. Does the tongue have a magenta hue? Are there any cracks at the corner of the lips? Does the patient have any rashes, dermatitis or inflamed bronchial mucosa? Is there alcohol abuse, trauma, use of antidepressants and oral contraceptives? All are indicative of an individual's need for riboflavin.

With a *niacinamide deficiency*, examine the tongue. Is it also swollen, inflamed or painful? Are there fissures on the lips? Is there any dermatitis or diarrhea? Is the patient experiencing depression, irritability or insomnia?

In a *pyridoxine (vitamin B6) deficiency*, does the tongue display a purplish color; is it painful and smooth? Are there fissures on the lips as opposed to the corners of the mouth? Is the throat swollen and sore? Does the patient complain of muscle twitches or a burning or tingling sensation in his hands and feet? Is there a history of carpal tunnel syndrome or restless leg syndrome? Has the patient been on hormone replacement therapy, birth control pills or the patch, all of which can lead to lower levels of vitamin B6 in the body? Does the patient have high blood homocysteine levels?

A *folate deficiency* presents greater diagnostic difficulty. Some deficiencies are not as visually apparent as others. If you suspect a folate deficiency, several relevant questions to ask your patients would be: Does he have cardiovascular problems (relating to high homocysteine levels), or is there a family history of cardiovascular problems? Is he anemic (specifically megaloblastic or macrocytic)? How is his short term memory? If your patient is female, has she recently been pregnant? Are organ meats eaten on a weekly basis? Are adequate amounts of dark, leafy green vegetables consumed daily?

Pernicious anemia is the most well known *vitamin B12 deficiency*. Fatigue and heart palpitations are early symptoms[26]. Neurological symptoms include numbness and tingling of the arms, hands, legs and feet, and appear in vitamin B12 deficiencies. Does the patient exhibit an unstable gait or movements? Is there depression or psychosis? Are there high homocysteine levels? Is he a vegetarian?

In an *iron deficiency*, besides the atrophy of taste buds, the tongue is pale in color. It may also be sore, and/or accompanied by angular stomatitis. Does the patient fatigue and become cold easily? Is their complexion pale? Look at the fingernails. Are they spoon shaped? Press on the nail. Does the pink color return within a few seconds to the nail bed after pressure has been released?

Thick, Yellow Coating on the Tongue and Digestion

A THICK, YELLOW COATING ON THE TONGUE INDICATES A digestive problem or constipation.

In a digestive problem, the recommended first approach is to heal the gastrointestinal tract with certain nutrients, along with the use of digestive enzymes. In this case, digestive enzymes are essential, because they help to completely digest the food, taking the burden from the digestive tract and allowing it to heal.

The lining of the gastrointestinal tract is made up of epithelial cells which require the same nutrient as the mucous membranes

---

26   Ibid., 194.

and skin. The nutrients necessary to promote healing and regeneration of epithelial tissue are the vitamin A, C and E complexes, trace minerals and amino acids. Recommend the patient eat chitterlings and tripe to speed the healing processes.

Add a demulcent such as aloe *(Aloe vera)*, slippery elm *(Ulmus spp.)*, licorice root *(Glycyrrhiza glabra)*, okra, marshmallow *(Althea officinalis)* or oats to the protocol. Demulcents are mucilaginous agents that sooth and heal an irritated and inflamed gastrointestinal tract by forming a protective coating over the mucosa. Again check for all contraindications and drug interactions before recommending adding herbs to your patient's protocol.

Thick, Yellow Coating on the Tongue and Constipation

THE OTHER CONDITION REFLECTIVE OF A YELLOW COATING on the tongue is constipation. A person with healthy digestive and intestinal function will have one to three bowel movements each day. Eating raw fruits and vegetables daily is essential for anyone with constipation to ensure they are getting enough fiber. Psyllium seed hulls are a good fiber substitute. Drinking six to eight glasses of pure water each day is also essential.

Most people know what foods move their bowels, whether it is prunes, sauerkraut, rhubarb, etc.

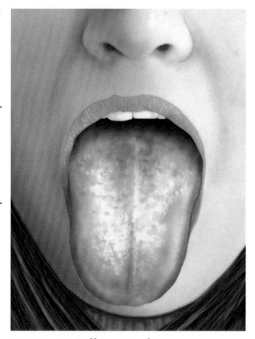

FIGURE 21. Yellow coated tongue

Have your patient consume these foods on a regular basis. Beets or beet greens are recommended to stimulate bile flow which will lubricate the stools. The mineral magnesium acts as a laxative. Blackstrap molasses is high in magnesium and other minerals. One teaspoon to two tablespoons per day will act as a food-based laxative. The herbs senna *(Cassia ssp.)*, aloe *(Aloe vera)* and cascara *(Rhamnus purshiana)* have traditionally been used as purgatives. Again check for contraindications and drug interactions before prescribing herbs.

Cannot Stick Tongue Out, Short Tongue or Trembling Tongue: Potential Cardiac or Stroke Patient

IN CHINESE TONGUE DIAGNOSIS, IF THE PATIENT CAN NOT stick out his tongue, if the tongue is short, tilted to one side, or when the tongue is extended it starts to tremble, can be symptoms indicative of a potential cardiac or stroke patient [27]. Immediate medical attention is advised, as well as nutritional support for the heart and vascular system. Think about it—it makes sense. The heart is a muscle. If the heart is weak, other muscles in the body will also be weak, including the muscles of the tongue.

For preclinical signs of a potential heart problem, look at the tip of the tongue. Does it appear to be thin, elongated, or red? Is the tip sore or does it burn? Are there any markings or forking? Are there lesions present? Another symptom commonly associated with a potential heart problem is discomfort in the chest that may radiate down the left arm. There may also be a faint or

---

27   Tsu-Tsair Chi, *Dr. Chi's Method of Fingernail and Tongue Analysis* (Chi Enterprises, 2002), 67-68.

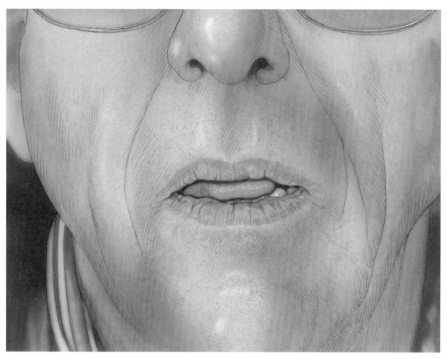

FIGURE 22. *Short tongue*

rapid pulse, palpitations, dizziness, fatigue, shortness of breath, headaches and a persistent cough.

The heart needs protein, a balance of saturated and unsaturated fats and an array of vitamins and minerals to function properly and be able to regenerate healthy, new heart tissue. The necessary vitamins and minerals are: the whole vitamin complexes B (including vitamin B4), C, E (including the E2 factors), F and G, along with the minerals calcium, iron, magnesium, potassium and phosphorous. Eating whole beef, pork, chicken, or turkey heart is also nutritionally beneficial. The herb hawthorne leaf (*Crataegus spp.*) is a cardio-tonic, cardio-protective and cardiac tropho-restorative. It should therefore be a consideration, as indicted, in

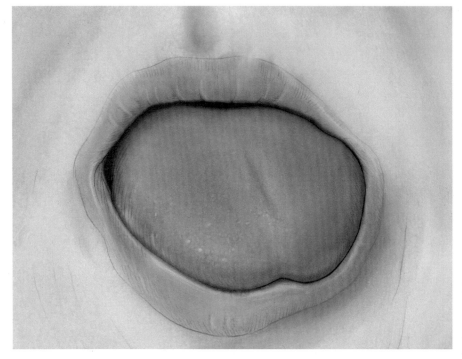

FIGURE 23. Forked and tilted tongue

cardiac cases. Be aware that the use of hawthorne may potentiate the action of some heart and blood pressure medications.

Besides tongue changes that can be early warning sign of a possible stroke, check for other indications of vascular problems. These would include gingivitis, spider veins, varicosities, ulcers, hemorrhoids or easy bruising.

Nutritionally support the vascular system with the whole vitamin C complex, rich in the vitamin P factor, which gives strength to the walls of the arteries, veins and capillaries. Foods high in rutin, quercetin and bioflavonoids such as buckwheat, red peppers, blueberries and the OPCs (oligomeric procyanidins) are high in the vitamin P factor.

The vitamin G complex may also be indicated for support in vascular cases. This nutrient has a vasodilating effect on the blood vessels and capillaries. In conjunction with vitamin G's lipotrophic property (of breaking up fat or cholesterol-causing atherosclerosis) and its nerve regenerating properties, it should be a considered nutrient for supporting stroke and high blood pressure patients.

Wheat germ oil is another supplement to consider using in a vascular support protocol. Besides being rich in the vitamin E complex, wheat germ oil increases the elasticity of the blood vessel walls. The berries of the hawthorne plant (*Crataegus spp.*) are rich in flavonoids and OPCs. They may be added to the protocol for additional support of the vascular system. It is important, when using herbs and nutrients with a cardiac patient, to have the prescribing physician regularly monitor heart medications.

Gingivitis

GINGIVITIS IS ANOTHER IMPORTANT NUTRITIONAL DEFI-ciency "tell-tale." As long as you are looking at the tongue and lips, glance at the gums. Red, swollen gingiva indicates a vitamin C complex deficiency. More specifically, it is a deficiency of the vitamin P factor of the whole vitamin C complex, which includes rutin, quercetin and other bioflavonoids.

Ascorbic acid alone will not heal and rebuild the gingiva[28]. Gingivitis is a capillary fragility disease and a symptom of pre-clinical scurvy. Left untreated, the collagen and connective tissue

28 Bicknell, and F. Prescott, *The Vitamins in Medicine* (New York: Grune and Stratton, 1953), 450.

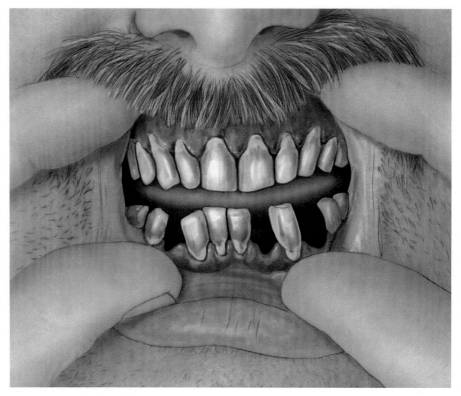

FIGURE 24. Gingivitis

breakdown in the gums and jaw can lead to periodontal destruction, increased tooth mobility and tooth exfoliation.

Other preclinical signs of vitamin C deficiencies are bruising easily, adrenal fatigue, frequent colds, influenzas and infections, spider veins, telangiectasis (facial road mapping) and corkscrew hairs.

The vitamin C complex is found in citrus fruits, berries, cherries, tomatoes, red peppers, raw mushrooms and potatoes. The anti-scorbutic phytochemicals of the vitamin P factor are found in red peppers, buckwheat, and citrus fruits, particularly in their rinds. It is best to eat these foods fresh and raw. It is important to

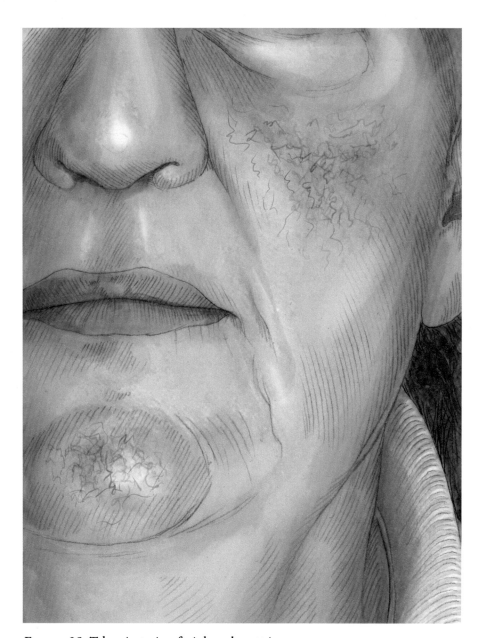

FIGURE 25. *Telangiectasis—facial road mapping*

note, vitamin C content is diminished by oxidation and the high temperatures of cooking. This fact emphasizes the importance for our health of including fresh, raw vegetables and fruit in our diets on a daily basis.

CHAPTER THREE

Fingernails

FINGERNAILS CAN BE A POTENT INDICATOR OF A PATIENT'S nutritional status. The nail bed contains many capillaries which bring nutrients to the nail root for the growth of the nail plate. Due to this abundance of capillaries and the accelerated rate at which the nails grow, they, like the tongue, reflect the health of the body. Healthy nail plates have a transparent pink color with a shiny luster and a smooth, even, arch shape. There should be lunulas on at least eight of the ten fingernails.

The nails, like the hair, are composed of dead cells that make up a protein called keratin. The hardness of the nail comes from the presence of sulfur in the amino acids that bind the keratin of the nails together. Between the layers of keratin are water and fat molecules which make the nails shiny and pliable. To have healthy nails the patient needs to consume, properly absorb and assimilate adequate amounts

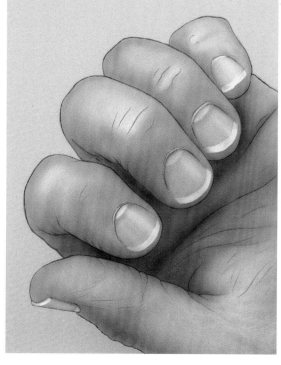

FIGURE 26. Healthy nails

of protein, essential fatty acids, trace minerals and pure water. Nails grow a tenth of a millimeter (0.1mm) a day; taking about six months to grow a whole new nail from root to tip. They are a virtual snapshot of the patient's health over the last six months. Abnormalities in the nails are associated with nutritional deficiencies, disease pathology and some pharmaceutical drugs. This text addresses only the deficiencies and diseases that have a nutritional basis that may be affecting the nails.

When examining your patient's fingernails, it is important to make sure you are looking at their real nails, not fake nails or extensions. There should be no polish on the nails, not even a clear polish. First, rule out any physical trauma or injury to the nail plate or nail bed. Patients will catch their fingertip in doors or drawers, or accidentally strike them with a hammer. The resulting marks from the injury do not reflect a nutritional deficiency or a disease state in the body.

Leukonychia

LEUKONYCHIA IS A TERM FOR WHITE SPOTS ON THE FINgernails. Traditionally, this is indicative of a zinc deficiency. However, this may also be caused by an excess consumption of refined sugars.

The mineral zinc is abundant in red meat, shellfish (oysters being exceptionally high in zinc), eggs, nuts, pumpkin seeds, legumes, molasses, brewer's yeast, rice bran and wheat germ. Zinc is necessary for proper growth and development, gene transcription and expression, fertility, wound healing, nerve transmission and

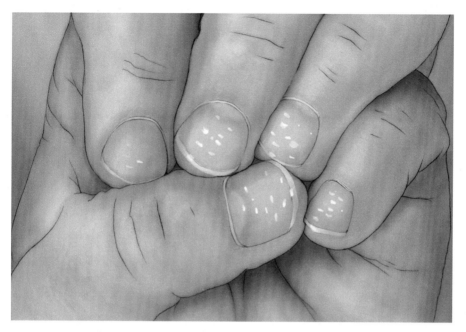

FIGURE 27. Leukonychia—white spots

optimum immune function[1]. Other signs of zinc deficiency include a weakened immune system, acne and rashes, reduced sense
of taste and smell, hair loss, stunted growth, late puberty, learning
difficulties and poor concentration in children, low sperm count
and infertility in both genders[2].

Augment the patient's diet with a zinc supplement that is
naturally chelated from a food source. For long-term zinc supplementation, use a zinc supplement that also contains naturally
occurring iron and copper. (The optimal ratio of copper to zinc
plasma or serum is 0.70 to 1.00.) It is important to honor the

---

1 Jane Higdon, *An Evidence Based Approach to Vitamins and Nutrition* (New
York: Thieme Publishing, 2003), 197.
2 Michael Zimmermann, *Macronutrients in Health and Disease* (New York:
Thieme Publishing, 2001), 63.

body's natural balance and interdependence of these nutrients when using nutraceuticals.

An over-consumption of refined sugars will lead to trace mineral deficiencies. In the refinement process, converting sugar cane, sugar beet, agave or corn to commercial sweeteners, trace minerals are stripped from the sugar molecule. When refined sugars are ingested, the body will actually pull these missing and needed nutrients from its own organs and tissues to utilize the refined sugar that is consumed if the needed nutrients are not present in the diet at the time of consumption. This can cause and compound other nutritional deficiencies, including zinc, calcium and thiamine. (Isn't it interesting that in addition to chromium, both zinc and B vitamins are necessary for the pancreas to produce the insulin necessary for the body to utilize sugar?) Nature packages whole, unprocessed foods with everything they need to be absorbed and utilized by the body. The commercial food industry, however, strips away the life-supporting elements and then adds back a few fraudulent chemical nutrients to our perishable foods to make them more readily transportable and give them a long shelf life.

That is why it is important to limit, if not completely eliminate refined sugars from our diets. There are many healthy alternatives that can be used as sweetening agents—agents that actually provide nutrients *to* the patient instead of depleting nutrients *from* them. With these natural sweetening agents, and a little time spent in the kitchen, it really is not difficult to eliminate refined sugars from our diets.

One of these natural alternatives is raw, dehydrated sugar

cane juice, which can be easily exchanged for table sugar. When using it in baked goods, 2/3 to 3/4 cups of raw, dehydrated sugar cane juice is equivalent to 1 cup refined sugar.

Honey is another good sugar substitute. Make sure the honey is raw and unfiltered. The vitamins, minerals, amino acids and antibacterial properties are destroyed in the refinement process. (Never use raw honey with an infant or toddler due to the possible presence of botulism spores in raw honey.)

Maple syrup is a flavorful alternative sweetener. It is high in malic acid and trace minerals. Grade B maple syrup is less refined than grade A, and therefore, higher in naturally occurring nutrients. When substituting liquid sweetener in baking recipes reduce the amount of natural sweetener by about one quarter and cut back on the other liquids in the recipe. It is easiest to substitute honey and maple syrup in pies and fruit desserts.

Blackstrap molasses is abundant in trace minerals. It can be easily and tastefully substituted in corn bread and pumpkin pie recipes. Stevia (*Stevia rebaudiana*) is natural herbal sweetening agent. It comes in a liquid form which dissolves readily in beverages.

Longitudinal Ridges

LONGITUDINAL RIDGES IN THE NAILS CAN BE A SIGN OF A vitamin F deficiency. Vitamin F is an old term for an array of essential fatty acids—linoleic acid, alpha-linolenic acid and arachidonic acid—which balanced together have a specific vitamin affect. Although the FDA does not presently recognize vitamin F, it is common used in nutrition books prior to the mid 1950s.

Vitamin F is necessary for healthy skin, hair and nails. It is needed for the proper function of the thyroid and prostate glands.

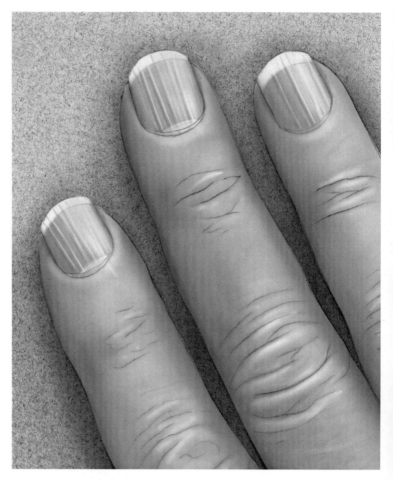

FIGURE 28. Longitudinal ridges

Besides its lubricating effect on synovial and cerebral spinal fluids, vitamin F assists in the transfer of calcium from the blood into the tissues[3]. Vitamin F will also raise blood iodine levels, making iodine more available to the thyroid gland and other tissues[4].

3 Royal Lee, "Food Integrity," *Conversations in Nutrition* (April, 1955), and Gary and Steve Null, *The Complete Handbook of Nutrition* (New York: Dell Publishing Co., 1972), 48.

4 "Vitamin F Perles," *Index of Product Bulletins (Milwaukee,WI: Vitamin Product Company, circa 1940's)*.

Weston A. Price, DDS, in his book *Nutrition and Physical Degeneration,* referred to vitamin F as the "X factor." The Weston A. Price Foundation is now referring to this nutrient as vitamin K2 [5].

Vitamin F is found in unrefined fish liver oils, egg yolks, cream, butter, fish eggs, fat-soluble chlorophyll, and fats from pastured animals fed on fresh green grasses, as well as raw nuts, flax seeds, avocados and their cold-pressed, unrefined oils.

Other signs of vitamin F deficiency are: calcium assimilation problems such as dry and itchy skin, muscle cramps and aches, propensity to sun and wind burn, a diminished second heart sound; also brittle nails, thyroid disease, enlarged prostate and dry and/or fallen hair. Vitamin F is available in supplement form as vitamin F complex, as X factor butters, or in unrefined or fermented cod liver oil products.

In the elderly patient, whose nails exhibit longitudinal ridges and who do not respond to vitamin F therapy look to and resolve any underlying heart problems.

Clubbing

CLUBBING IS A TERM USED TO DESCRIBE NAILS THAT HAVE a pronounced convex curve. To determine if a patient has clubbed nails, use the *Schamroth sign.* It defines clubbing, as "the obliteration of the normal diamond-shaped space at the proximal end of the nail when the distal phalanges are opposed."[6] In other words, when you put the fingers together on the knuckle sides, there

5 Chris Masterjohn, "On the Trail of the Illusive X Factor," *Wise Traditions,* Vol. 8, No.1 (Spring, 2007), 14-32.
6 Robert S. Fawcett, Sean Lanford, Daniel L. Stulberg, "Nail Abnormalities: Clues to System Disease," *American Family Physician* (March 15, 2004).

should be a diamond shape hole between the knuckle and the tip of the fingernail. In clubbing of the fingernails, there will be an open triangular wedge; the tips of the nails do not touch.

Clubbing is associated with such conditions as pulmonary, heart or liver disease, celiac disease and inflammatory bowel. In the case of pulmonary or heart disease, the change in the nail plate is due to the depletion of oxygen in the blood which is the result of the associated lung or heart dysfunction.

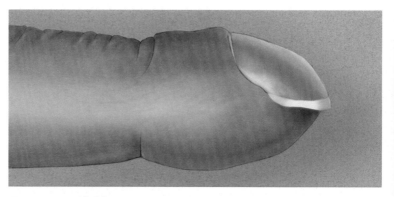

Figure 29. Clubbing

In all causes of clubbing, first check for and treat any blood anemia that may be the cause of, or exacerbating, low blood oxygen levels. Hemoglobin carries oxygen in the blood[7]. It is important that the patient has adequate size and density of red blood cells. Iron and copper are active in the formation of hemoglobin. Refer to Chapter Two—*Pale Tongue and Iron Deficiency*—for the nutritional support of an anemic patient.

The whole vitamin C complex increases the oxygen-carrying

7 Arthur C. Guyton, *Text Book of Medical Physiology* (Philadelphia, PA W.B. Saunders Co., 1986), 496.

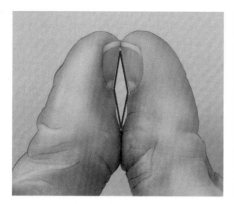 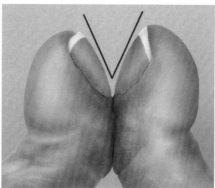

FIGURE 30. Schamroth's sign—normal   *FIGURE 31. Schamroth's sign—clubbing*

capacity of the blood[8]. Tyrosinase, a copper-containing enzyme, is the trace mineral activator of the whole vitamin C complex. Tyrosinase acts as an enzyme in the transport of oxygen from the lungs into the blood[9]. Copper is found in foods rich in vitamin C. Other food sources of copper include raw mushrooms, almonds, liver, egg yolks, shrimp, oysters, dried beans and lentils.

The whole vitamin E complex conserves oxygen in the blood[10]. Royal Lee, DDS, has specifically identified the vitamin E2 component of the vitamin E complex to be the oxygen-conserving factor of blood which helps enable the delivery of oxygen from the blood into the tissues. He demonstrated this with the use of the endocardiograph.

Wheat germ, beef heart and cold-pressed, unrefined oil from the germs of grains and seeds, particularly wheat germ oil, are high in this oxygen-saving factor. The vitamin E2 factor is

8 Judith A. DeCava, *The Real Truth About Vitamins and Antioxidants* (Columbus, GA: Brentwood Academic Press, 1996), 183, 195.
9 Ibid., 199.
10 Nutrition Research Inc., *Nutrition Almanac* (McGraw-Hill Book Co., USA, 1975), 52.

especially beneficial for patients with angina or emphysema; and those individuals who live, vacation or play at high altitude and feel its effect.

In cases of emphysema, start by nutritionally supporting the patient's lungs and adrenal glands. The adrenals are the endocrine glands that rule over lung function. Epinephrine and norepinephrine affect lung motility by increasing lung ventilation[11]. For resolution of any long-term lung condition it is essential to also support the adrenal glands.

An easy-to-perform test for adrenal insufficiency is the *Ragland's Test for Hypo-Adrenal Function*. D.C. Ragland, M.D., wrote a prize winning paper, "The Postural Blood Pressure Method of Evaluating Adrenal Hypofunction," in 1920, which explains his technique for measuring the adrenals ability to compensate for the hydrostatic effects of gravity.

When the body is in a horizontal position, there is less effect of gravity and less pressure is needed to get blood to the brain, resulting in a slight decrease in the blood pressure. When the individual stands or sits up quickly, the blood pressure increases to counter the effects of gravity and keeps blood flowing to the brain. The nerves in the splanchnic veins constrict to compensate for this effect of gravity. The splanchnic nerves are under the control of the adrenal glands. Hence, if the splanchnic nerve tone is weak, the adrenal glands are weak. In an individual with sufficient adrenal function, the systolic blood pressure should be 4 to 10 mm. higher in the erect position than in a recumbent position. If

---

11 Stefan Silbernagl and Florian Lang, *Color Atlas of Pathophysiology* (New York: Thieme Publishing, 2000), 82.

the patient's blood pressure remains the same or decreases upon standing, it is indicative of a possible hypoadrenia case. Also, the degree of the drop in the blood pressure is directly proportional to the degree of hypoadrenia[12].

To perform Dr. Ragland's screen-test for adrenal hypofunction, have the patient lie in a recumbent position. Using a blood pressure cuff around the bicep muscle, take the systolic blood pressure reading and record. Leave the blood pressure cuff on the patient's upper arm and pump it up again. Then have the patient stand and immediately take another blood pressure reading and record. If you begin pumping the cuff up after the patient stands, you give the body time to adapt and will not have an accurate test result. The systolic blood pressure should increase 4 to 10 mm. in the standing position from the recumbent position. Immediately repeat the test a second time for the most accurate results.

The adrenal glands require the vitamin C and G complexes, copper, calcium, potassium, sodium, manganese, iron, tyrosine, phenylalanine and cholesterol for hormone synthesis and proper function. The whole vitamin C complex is essential to adrenal function and prevents the oxidation of its hormones. Adrenal glandular products are helpful additions in resolving many adrenal and pulmonary disorders. Herbal adrenal adaptogens such as withania root (*Withania somnifera*), Siberian ginseng root (*Eleutherococcus senticosus*), Korean ginseng root (*Panax ginseng*) and astragalus root (*Astragalus membranaceus*) are useful when rebuilding the adrenal glands' health and function. Remember,

---

12 D.C. Ragland, "The Postural Blood Pressure Method of Evaluating Adrenal Hypofunction," (Los Angeles, CA, 1920).

when using herbs, to check for any contraindications and drug interactions.

Protocols for the emphysema patient need to focus on nourishing the alveoli of the lungs. The alveoli require whole vitamin A and C complexes and trace minerals for proper functioning and regeneration. Foods rich in both vitamin C and provitamin A include fresh oranges, red grapefruits, tangerines, cranberries, gooseberries, papayas, sweet potatoes, yellow squash, turnip greens, peppers, kale, cabbage, nettle *(Urtica spp.)* and parsley *(Petroselinum crispum)*. Carotenoids and carotenes are considered provitamin A. They are the substances responsible for the yellow and orange pigments in fruits and vegetables. Provitamin A is converted into vitamin A (retinol) in the enterocytes lining the intestinal walls in the presence of fat. Advise your patients to put a little pat of butter or a drizzle of olive oil on their vegetables before eating them. The addition of a lung glandular supplement can be advantageous to restoring proper lung function and health.

For clubbing associated with heart disease, nutritionally support the heart with the vitamin B, E and G complexes. Wheat germ oil is a potent source of the whole vitamin E complex, including the vitamin F and vitamin E2 factors. Wheat germ oil goes rancid easily so be careful to store it properly. It is also available in hermetically sealed perles as a supplement. Eating wheat germ will additionally provide the protein the heart needs. Nutritional yeasts are an excellent source of vitamin B and G complexes. Calcium and potassium are essential to proper heart function. These essential minerals are found abundantly in kelp, alfalfa, parsley *(Petroselinum crispum)*, broccoli, Swiss chard, mustard, collards and dandelion greens. Have the patient include in their diet plenty of naturally raised, cooked beef, pork, lamb, chicken, or turkey heart. The heart contains vitamin B4—the anti-paralysis factor—which will innervate the heart muscle. If the patient is unwilling to eat heart, recommend a heart glandular supplement.

When the clubbing is associated with liver disease, nourish the liver with the fat-soluble vitamins A, D and E. Cod liver oil and fat-soluble chlorophyll are a good source of these nutrients. If the patient belches when ingesting nutritionally rich oils or fats, it is an indication of insufficient bile production or flow. Eating or juicing raw beets, beet leaves and spinach provide rich sources of betaine which thins the bile by converting blood fat to glycogen. If the patient's gallbladder has been removed, give them a bile salt supplement to take with meals to ensure digestion and assimilation of their dietary fats and fat-soluble vitamins.

Blackstrap molasses is an excellent source of the trace minerals necessary for the liver's health and function. Eating naturally raised chicken, beef or pork liver is also beneficial. Again, if the patient is adverse to this, add a liver glandular supplement to their protocol.

Celiac patients with clubbed fingernails need to remove grains and cereals from their diet. Gluten is a protein found in the endosperm of grains. It is the substance in grains that allows flour to leaven. A celiac patient is gluten intolerant; eating gluten triggers an immune response in the intestinal mucosa. In some celiac patients, this response will cause pathological changes that can damage the intestines causing a reduction in their absorption of nutrients. In a severe allergic reaction to gluten, this immune response will flood the blood stream with lymphocytes. Improvement occurs when grains high in gluten such as wheat, rye, barley, and oats are eliminated from the patient's diet.

In addition to the elimination of grain and flour products, it is important to add a digestive aid that is high in enzymes and hydrochloric acid. This will enable the stomach to fully digest food, in particular protein. It will also reduce the stress from the intestines, requiring them to do less digestive work, giving them an opportunity to heal.

As mentioned above, supplementation of bile salts may be required. Bile is essential to help digest and utilize fat that often appears in the celiac patient's stools. Furthermore, bile heals the intestinal mucosa.

Demulcents, such as okra, aloe (*Aloe vera*), comfrey (*Symphytum officinalis*) (if no history of cancer), marshmallow root (*Althea officinalis*), licorice root (*Glycyrrhiza glabra*) (if there is no high blood pressure or edema), or slippery elm (*Ulmus spp.*) are nourishing and sooth the irritated and inflamed intestinal lining.

Whole vitamin A and C complexes are needed to support the healing of the mucous membranes of the intestines. They have natural anti-inflammatory properties as well. Vitamin C complex is necessary for collagen regeneration to repair intestinal permeability which allows undigested protein to pass into the blood stream, initiating an antigen-antibody immune response. This is also known as the "Leaky Gut Syndrome." A vitamin A and C supplement may be needed adjunctively for the patient who is unable or unwilling to add the foods high in these nutrients into their diet.

Fermented foods should be included in the diet of the celiac patient. These foods will help re-establish the intestinal flora for optimal digestion and absorption of carbohydrates and other nutrients. Suggested fermented foods include yogurt, kefir, miso, tempeh, sauerkraut, kimchi, pickles and kvas. An acidophilus and bifidus, or a mycelium yeast supplement may be substituted or used in tandem.

It will take about six months to repair the damage done to the intestine by the disease. After the intestines are healed, patients may tolerate starches low in gluten such as rice, millet, buckwheat, farro, corn, amaranth and quinoa. These patients may require long-term use of digestive enzymes.

With clubbing associated with inflammatory bowel, Crohn's disease and ulcerative colitis look for a bacterial, viral, parasitic, food allergy/sensitivity or yeast involvement exacerbating the inflammatory process. The aforementioned conditions have similar symptoms and pathology occurring in varying degrees in different parts of the intestines.

These diseases are practically nonexistent in cultures that still eat their primitive diet[13]. They ae diseases of the intestines brought on by a diet of refined and devitalized, commercial foods. Therefore, a diet of well cooked and ripened, but unprocessed, unrefined foods should be eaten until the patient is asymptomatic. Raw foods and fiber will aggravate these conditions until the

---

13 Russell B. Marz, *Medical Nutrition From Marz*, 2nd Edition (Portland, Oregon: Omni-Press, 1999), 377.

intestines are healed. However, after repair, the addition of these foods is essential to long-term remission and restoration of the intestines.

Each case must be treated individually due to the many contributing factors to these intestinal disorders. Address and correct all of the patient's underlying involvements. It is important to make the patient comfortable by alleviating their symptoms. Some of those symptoms include diarrhea, bloody stools, infection, fever, inflammation, abdominal cramping, weight loss and malnutrition. Look for and rectify any emotional component which may be adding to their physical symptoms. Such a component can manifest itself as stress, anxiety and/or depression, which can be highly detrimental to the ultimate recovery of the patient.

Begin with an elimination diet; eliminate the offending foods that are eliciting allergic responses. The most common culprits are wheat, corn, soy pasteurized dairy and food additives. Also omit spicy, hot foods that irritate the gastrointestinal lining. Caffeine and alcohol should be temporarily eliminated. In severe cases, the patient may have to limit their diet warm vegetable and bone broths for the first two weeks. Ideally, the patient should drink pure spring or filtered water, free of fluoride and chlorine.

The initial diet should consist of warm vegetable, fish and meat broths. These are easily digestible and supply much-needed nutrients to the patient. Incorporate fresh, ripe bananas, pears, and peaches, well-cooked, fresh vegetables and fresh, raw vegetable juices.

Raw cabbage juice contains allantoin and vitamin U, which

cleanses and heals the mucous membranes of the intestinal tract. Raw, fresh, green, leafy vegetable juice contains chlorophyll, a cell proliferator that sooths and repairs the gastrointestinal lining. Chlorophyll also contains vitamin K which will staunch any intestinal bleeding by promoting the synthesis of prothrombin. A fat-soluble chlorophyll supplement, best taken on an empty stomach, may be used in adjunct.

If the patient does not react to the above dietary changes, add fish and light animal protein, followed by well-cooked oats, rice, millet or quinoa. When the intestines are healed, reintroduce red meat, beans and other grains into the diet. Continue to eliminate any and all foods that elicit an allergic response. The food combining diet also works well for these intestinal cases. Counsel the patient on a life-long diet change, eliminating processed and refined foods (from a box or a can) and eating fresh and wholesome foods that are high in fiber and nutrients.

Nutritionally support the restoration and health of the intestinal lining as you would with celiac disease, using foods and supplements high in the whole vitamins A, C and P complexes, trace minerals and amino acids. Vitamin A complex is found abundantly in fish liver oil, kidneys, liver, butter and cream. Carrots and leafy green vegetables (beet greens, spinach, kale and broccoli) contain carotene, a provitamin A, which a healthy person can convert into vitamin A. The vitamin C complex is abundant in citrus fruits, berries, cherries, tomatoes, red peppers, raw mushrooms and potatoes. Vitamin P is also known as the bioflavonoid component of the vitamin C complex, which includse rutin, quercetin, herpseridin, myrecetin, nobiletin and tangeritin.

They are the component of the vitamin C complex necessary for collagen production and strengthening the vascular walls. These anti-scorbutic phytochemicals are found in red peppers, buckwheat, citrus fruit (abundantly in the rinds), blueberries and the OPCs (oligomeric procyanidins).

The use of a demulcent, such as okra, aloe (*Aloe vera*), marshmallow root (*Althea officinalis)* or slippery elm (*Ulmus spp.*), will work to sooth and restore the inflamed intestinal mucosa. The patient will also require digestive enzymes, preferably with hydrochloric acid, at each meal. This will maximize digestion of the food in the stomach before it enters the compromised intestines. As with all gastro-intestinal disorders it is important to have the patient incorporate fermented foods into their diet. These probiotic foods (yogurt, kefir, buttermilk, etc.) will help re-establish the optimal intestinal pH and friendly bacteria. With a dairy allergy or vegan patient, recommend incorporating fermented vegetable such as tempeh, miso, sauerkraut, pickles, etc. into their diet. An acidophilus or mycelium yeast supplement may also be used.

If there is a parasitic involvement, consider using digestive enzymes such as amylase, lipase and cellulose, taken on an empty stomach to digest the parasites. Herbs such as garlic (*Allium sativa*), wormwood (*Artemisia absinthium*) and black walnut (*Juglans nigra*) hulls are also effective for eradicating a parasitic infection. However, use them cautiously for they may further irritate the intestinal lining. Remember to check for all contraindications and interactions before prescribing an herbal remedy.

Koilonychia

KOILONYCHIA, OR SPOON NAILS, IS A DYSTROPHY OF THE

fingernails. The nails actually lose their natural slight convex curve and turn concave instead. They become thin, upturned, and brittle; taking on the shape of a spoon. Hence the term "spoon" nails. This condition is associated with blood iron disorders such an anemia or hemochromatosis.

Anemia can be caused by too little iron in the blood; conversely, hemochromatosis is too much iron in the blood. Similar symptoms can occur from a nutrient deficiency as well as a

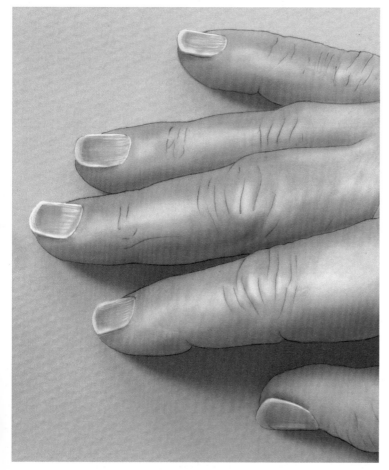

FIGURE 32. Koilonychia—spoon nails

nutrient overload. Spoon nails is one example. Beeturia, (red tinted urine after ingesting beets) is another sign of either iron deficiency or hemochromatosis.

The best bioavailable food sources of iron include red meat, liver and organ meats, fish, oysters and poultry. These food sources contain heme iron which is more readily absorbed than the non-heme source. Less bioavailable food sources include spinach and dark, leafy green vegetables, egg yolks and blackstrap molasses. If using an iron supplement, recommend one from a liver source which will also contain naturally occurring folate and vitamin B12. Remember folate is needed to produce red blood cells in the long bones of the body and vitamin B12 is necessary to mature them. Please refer back to the section on *pale tongue* in Chapter Two for more details on nutritional support necessary to reverse iron deficiency anemia.

Besides reducing intake of dietary iron, the nutritional support of a hemochromatosis patient should be aimed at optimizing the body's ability to drive the excess iron in the blood into the muscle where it is stored and utilized as myoglobin.

It is imperative not to use an ascorbic acid supplement for a patient with hemochromatosis. Ascorbic acid will increase the body's ability to absorb iron from the intestines and will contribute to the iron overload. On the other hand, the whole vitamin C complex will assist hemoglobin's function of carrying iron in the blood. Therefore recommend a whole food, vitamin C complex supplement or foods high in vitamin C. Again, foods high in vitamin C complex include fresh, raw, citrus fruits, berries, cherries, tomatoes, red peppers, potatoes and mushrooms.

The addition of copper is essential in the support of hemochromatosis. An often overlooked consideration when working with mineral imbalances in the body is to use their related minerals to keep the blood values in homeostasis. Please refer to the *Mineral Relationship Chart* in the Appendix. Copper helps the body utilize the iron. Copper-containing enzymes are necessary for the transport of iron[14]. Therefore the addition of copper will suppress iron in the blood by transporting it where it is needed for utilization. Foods high in copper are mushrooms, almonds, egg yolks, shrimp, dried beans and peas. If using a supplement with trace minerals, keep in mind that elemental minerals are handled differently in the body than minerals found in whole foods. They are needed in trace amounts. Be careful not to over dose them.

Phosphorous is another mineral to add to the nutritional support of a hemochromatosis patient because phosphorous depresses iron levels. Phosphorous also nourishes the sympathetic nervous system. The sympathetic nervous system impacts how quickly the body utilizes iron. Phosphorous deficiencies are also related to calcium metabolism and precipitation problems. A normal blood ratio should be 10 parts calcium to 4 parts phosphorous.

Signs of this imbalance include elevated blood calcium, high blood viscosity, calcium stones, spurring and tartar build up on teeth. The best food sources of phosphorous are meat, fish, eggs, seeds, fresh ground grains and bones. Therapeutically recommend

---

14 Jane Higdon, *An Evidence Base Approach to Vitamins and Nutrition* (New York: Thieme Publishing, 2003), 116.

a natural orthophosphoric acid supplement. Mix the liquid in a little water, tea or juice to ingest. Phosphorus can also increase heart rate so dose accordingly. Because of these actions the use of a phosphoric acid supplement is contraindicated in tachycardia and with pharmaceutical blood thinners.

Onychocryptosis

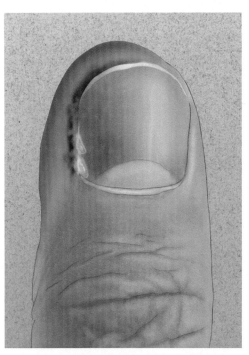

INGROWN NAILS OR ONY-chocryptosis is very painful. To prevent ingrown nails, recommend the patient trim their nails straight across, instead of curved. When dealing with ingrown toenails, make sure the patient's shoes and socks are fitted properly. Shoes that are too tight can cause an ingrown toenail. It is imperative for the patient to keep the area around the ingrown nail clean at all times to reduce the risk of an infection.

FIGURE 33. Onychocryptosis—ingrown nails

While inflamed, if at all possible, trim the ingrown nail away from the skin. Apply a *fat-soluble* chlorophyll ointment and cover with a band aid. Have the patient repeat this every day, keeping the affected area covered until the infection has cleared. It usually will take a few days to two weeks for complete resolution.

Chlorophyll, or plant blood, is high in vitamins E, F, K and provitamin A. This makes it an excellent healing and an anti-scarring agent for the epithelial tissue. The vitamin K provides blood clotting factors to help staunch bleeding. It is also a natural cleansing and purifying agent. Be aware that *water-soluble* chlorophyll will not contain these fat-soluble vitamins. No medicine cabinet should be without a jar of this topical salve. Chlorophyll will stain fabrics, so keep the affected area well covered. Rubbing alcohol will remove any residual green color from the skin.

Onychomycosis

ONYCHOMYCOSIS OR FUNGUS OF THE NAILS CAN OCCUR IN either the finger or toenails. It can be very embarrassing. Women who have this plight cannot get pedicures, and they rarely wear sandals or open-toe shoes. This topical infection is indicative of a systemic fungal infection which needs to be nutritionally addressed as well. Resolution of this condition will take time and effort by a conscious patient along with dietary and hygiene changes.

Have the patient add fermented foods to their diet. Some of these foods include yogurt, kefir, miso, tempeh, sauerkraut, kimchi, pickles and kvas. Restrict the intake of refined carbohydrates and sugars. Consider as adjunct to the diet a mycelium yeast or acidophilus and bifidus bacteria supplement. Remember, mycelium yeast will convert any sugar or carbohydrate in the diet to lactic acid.

Acidophilus bacteria, found in yogurt and kefir, prefers to convert lactose, or milk sugar, into lactic acid. Lactic acid changes the pH in the large intestines and bowel to its natural acid state; an environment in which the healthy beneficial flora can

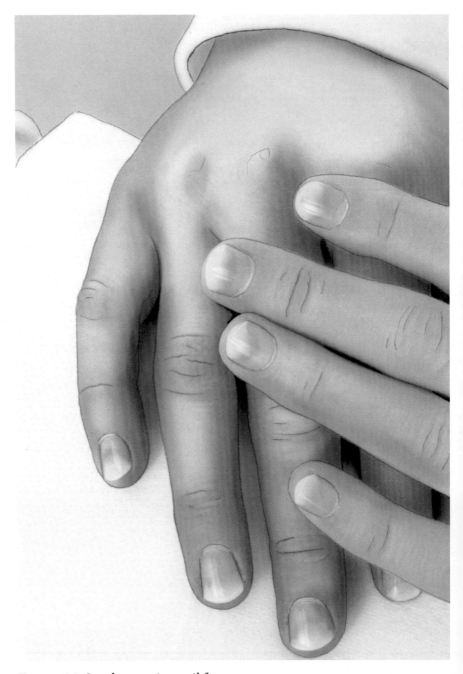

FIGURE 34. Onychomycosis—nail fungus

proliferate and thrive, starving out the Candida and fungal infections. It is important to inform the patient they may experience bowel discomfort, gas, bloating, belching and flatulence for a couple of weeks while the flora is re-establishing. Please refer back to *Geographic Tongue* in the previous chapter for more information on fungal/yeast infections.

An imperative part of this healing regimen is to attend to the topical fungal infection of the nail. Adjunctive application of white iodine to the effective area is beneficial. It must be applied twice daily, continually without interruption, to the involved nails and surrounding cuticle area until the infection is resolved. Other daily topical recommendations of tea tree oil, white vinegar and even Vick's Vapor Rub have traditionally been used successfully to aid in the resolution of this condition.

Have the patient soak the effective area in a warm pau d'arco *(Tabebuia impetiginosa)* or cat's claw (*Uncaria tomentosa*) infusion once a day. It is soothing and will fight the infection topically. These herbs may also be taken internally to reconcile the systemic fungal infection.

Lack of Lunulas

THE LUNULA IS THE CRESCENT MOON SHAPED LIGHT AREA at the base of the nail, above the cuticle. There should be lunulas on at least eight of the 10 fingernails. Less than eight lunulas on the fingernails can be an indication of low cellular oxygen levels or poor circulation[15]. The use of high potency antioxidant

---

15 Tsu-Tsair Chi, *Dr. Chi's Method of Fingernail and Tongue Analysis* (Chi Enterprises, 2002), 42,110.

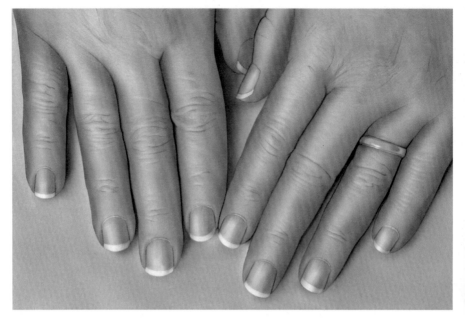

FIGURE 35. Lack of lunulas

supplements has been clinically observed to cause or exacerbate this condition.

Hemoglobin, with the assistance of the vitamin C complex, carries oxygen in the blood[16]. Iron is essential for the formation of hemoglobin. The best bioavailable food sources of iron include red meat, liver and organ meats, fish, oysters and poultry. Less bioavailable food sources include spinach and dark, leafy green vegetables, egg yolks and blackstrap molasses. Therapeutically, recommend an iron supplement from a liver or food source.

Vitamin C complex is found abundantly in citrus fruits, berries, cherries, tomatoes, red peppers, raw mushrooms and potatoes. Vitamin C in fruits and vegetables starts to diminish the

16 Judith A. DeCava, *The Real Truth About Vitamins and Antioxidants* (Columbus, GA: Brentwood Academic Press, 1996), 183.

moment they are picked. Their vitamin C content is further reduced by oxidation (exposure to air) and the high temperatures
of cooking. So it is best to eat these foods fresh and raw. If the
patient does not eat adequate amounts of produce (five to nine
servings/day) augment their diet with a food-based vitamin C
supplement.

The whole vitamin E complex conserves oxygen in the blood[17].
Wheat germ, beef heart and cold-pressed, unrefined oil from the
germs of grains and seeds, particularly wheat germ oil, are high
in the vitamin E's oxygen-conserving factor. Wheat germ oil de-
grades quickly in the presence of heat, light and air, diminishing
its valuable vitamin E components. Like flax seed oil, it requires
extra care when handling and storing it. Therapeutically, use
wheat germ oil or a food-based vitamin E supplement.

Remove any high dose synthetic or crystalline vitamin extract
(ascorbic acid, tocopherols, beta carotene) from the patient's nutritional protocol. These are high in antioxidants. In recent studies, consumption of these extracts increased cancer rates rather
than gave protection from certain cancers[18]. The use of high dose
antioxidants supplements have been shown to prevent oxygen
from working properly within the cell. They seem to inhibit the
metabolism of oxygen and oxygen-dependant reactions includ-

---

17 Nutrition Research Inc., *Nutrition Almanac* (McGraw-Hill Book Co.,
USA, 1975), 52.
18 Isabelle Bairati, François Meyer, Michel Gélinas, André Fortin, Abdenour
Nabid, François Brochet, Jean-Philippe Mercier, Bernard Têtu, François
Harel, Benoît, Mâsse, Éric Vigneault, Sylvie Vass, Pierre del Vecchio, and
Jean Roy, "A Random Trial of Antioxidant Vitamins to Prevent Second
Primary Cancers in Head and Neck Cancer Patients," *Journal of the National
Cancer Inst* (2005) 97, 481-488.

ing enzymes, coenzymes, polypeptides and other mitochondrial oxidative reactions in the body[19].

A better way to supply antioxidants is to eat adequate amounts of fresh foods and herbs in the diet. This will provide enough antioxidants material to fight free-radical pathology and contribute to antioxidant enzyme production without the detrimental effects of an overload. Foods and herbs rich in naturally occurring antioxidants include strawberries, blackberries, cranberries, raspberries, blueberries, walnuts, artichokes, cloves (*Eugenia aromatic*), green tea and rosemary (*Rosmarinus officinalis*).

Nutritional support to increase the blood flow and address the circulation involvement in lack of lunulas should include vitamin G, un-coded ribonucleic acid and the mineral phosphorus. The vitamin G factors of the B vitamin complex have vasodilating properties, increasing the diameter of the blood vessels allowing blood to flow more readily through the vessels. The vitamin G factors include vitamins B2, B3, B6, choline, inositol, folate and biotin. These B vitamin components are insoluble in alcohol. The vitamin G factors are also nerve relaxing, nerve regenerating and lipotrophic.

Raw milk, liver, organ meats, red meat, nutritional yeast, blackstrap molasses, egg yolks, and green, leafy vegetables are some of the foods abundant in these vitamin G factors. Therapeutically recommend a food-based vitamin B complex high in these G factors. For more information about these vitamin G

---

19 Rudolf I. Salganik, Craig D. Albright, Jerolyn Rodgers, John Kim, Steven H. Zeisel. Mikhail S. Sivashinskiy, and Terry A. Van Dyke, "Dietary Antioxidant Depletion: Enhancement of Tumor Apoptosis and Inhibition of Brain Tumor Growth in Transgenic Mice," *Carcinogenesis* (2000) 21(5), 909-914.

factors, please refer to the section on *Pellagra* in the Chapter Two, The Tongue, under *Niacinamide deficiency*.

Un-coded ribonucleic acid (RNA) is a safe nutrient that thins the blood without damaging the blood vessel or the gastric mucosal lining. RNA is a template to make proteins for the repair and regeneration of tissue. Amino acids bind to RNA in the blood. The energy generated by that biochemical reaction heats, hence thins, the blood, increasing the circulation. It is also touted as an anti-aging nutrient. RNA is found abundantly in fish, especially sardines, as well as organ meats, chlorella and nutritional yeasts. Un-coded ribonucleic acid is also available in a supplement form.

Phosphorous will improve circulation by lowering blood viscosity. Phosphorous binds with calcium in the blood to form calcium phosphate. Calcium phosphate is readily transferred from the blood into the bone. The reduction of calcium will lower blood viscosity and thin the blood. Phosphorous will also reduce calcium deposits and plaqueing in the blood vessels, muscles and on the bones and teeth. Phosphorous nourishes and stimulates the sympathetic nervous system. It will also increase heart rate. Orthophosphoric acid is available as a food supplement. When therapeutically using phosphoric acid long term, it is best to recommend a calcium supplement (taken at a different time of day than the phosphorus) to prevent an imbalance in the calcium-to-phosphorus ratio. The use of a phosphoric acid supplement is contraindicated with a tachycardia patient or with a patient that is on a pharmaceutical blood thinner.

Some herbs to consider for treatment of lack of lunulas are ginkgo and cayenne pepper. Ginkgo (*Ginkgo biloba*) leaf increases peripheral circulation to the limbs and brain[20] and increases oxygenation of tissue[21]. Cayenne pepper (*Capsicum spp.*) has a warming effect on the body. It has traditionally been used to improve the circulation of blood, especially gustatory and peripheral circulation. Again, check for any contraindications and drug interactions before recommending herbal supplementation.

High dosages of tocopherols or vitamin E will also thin the blood. Because it is an antioxidant and a crystalline or synthetic extract of a whole vitamin complex it is not a recommended first option over the above-mentioned nutritional and herbal support.

Always look for and treat a heart involvement in any circulation problem. Refer to Chapter One for nutritional support of the heart. Remember, exercise is a great way to increase oxygenation and circulation of both the blood and the lymph.

Periungual Hemorrhaging

PERIUNGUAL HEMORRHAGING IS A MULTIPLE SPLINTER HEMorrhaging of the nail bed, forming a red crescent around the base of the cuticle and at the distal end under the nail plate. Periungual hemorrhaging is actually a sign of scurvy[22]. Scurvy is a severe vita-

---

20 Sharon Tilgner, *Herbal Medicine from the Heart of the Earth* (Creswell, OR: Wise Acre Press, Inc., 1999), 67.
21 S. Mills and K. Bone, *Principal and Practices of Phytotherapy* (New York: Churchill Livingstone, 2000), 404.
22 F. Bicknell, and F. Prescott, *The Vitamins in Medicine* (New York: Grune and Stratton, 1953), 450.

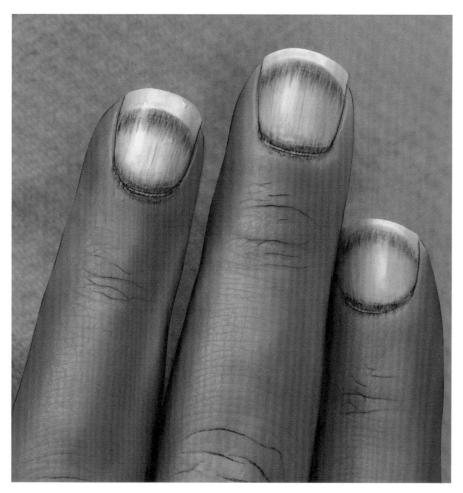

FIGURE 36. Periungual hemorrhaging

min C deficiency disease. It can be due to the insufficient intake of vitamin C rich foods in the diet (raw fruits and vegetables) or the inability to absorb and utilize vitamin C from food in the diet.

Scurvy has literally plagued humanity since ancient times. Scurvy was the demise of many sailors prior to James Lind, who in 1747, discovered that eating citrus fruits could cure and prevent scurvy. His recommendations led the English Royal Navy to serve citrus fruits to all their sailors on long sea voyages. It was the introduction of the potato into Western Europe that halted the yearly epidemic of scurvy that occurred at the end of every winter season due to the lack of fresh fruits and vegetables. Both citrus fruits and potatoes are rich in vitamin C. Freshly brewed beer, preserved fruits and the herb nettle (*Urtica spp.*) have also historically been consumed to ward off the devastating effects of scurvy.

Without adequate amounts of vitamin C the body cannot synthesize or repair collagen. Collagen is an essential component of connective tissue. Connective tissue is the foundation for all bone, dentin, cartilage, epithelial tissue and the blood vessel walls. Unlike other nutrients, such as certain B vitamins and vitamin K, vitamin C cannot be manufactured by the human body. Consuming foods containing this vitamin is essential for health and survival.

In the early stages of scurvy, the patient complains of: pains in the bones, muscles and joints; weakness and fatigue upon exertion; breathlessness; heart palpitations; a feeling of being tired and anorexia. In advancing cases the patient wants to sit rather than stand or walk. When the patient does stand or walk they will flex their legs due to the breakdown of their cartilage. Next to occur are the vascular fragility aspects of scurvy including periungual and perifollicular hemorrhages, corkscrew hairs, gingivitis, aneurisms, bleeding ulcers, telangiectasis (facial road mapping) and spider veins. The vascular integrity insufficiency of scurvy is a combined deficiency of ascorbic acid (vitamin C) and its related compound vitamin P (bioflavonoids)[23]. Left untreated, scurvy

---

23 Ibid., 449-450.

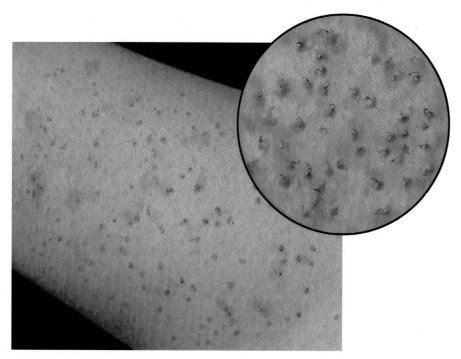

FIGURE 37. Corkscrew hairs

will eventually lead to death. The afore-mentioned conditions should be considered as preclinical scurvy. The cartilage breakdown can be correlated with many of today's arthritic conditions. This is why it is important to know the signs and symptoms and address underlying nutritional deficiencies which may be occurring in your patients.

Ingesting an isolated ascorbic acid $(C_6H_8O_6)$ supplement can potentially create other deficiencies in the body. Ascorbic acid has become the marker for vitamin C activity in the body and is now considered to be vitamin C by the FDA. As an antioxidant, ascorbic acid is the protecting or preserving factor of the whole vitamin C complex. It is there to protect the other valuable active enzymatic components of the whole vitamin C complex naturally occurring in our foods, compounds that are capable of changing body physiology. In other words, ascorbic acid is only a fraction of the vitamin C molecule that is found naturally occurring in foods.

Vitamins from food are biological complexes—protein in nature—consisting of enzymes, coenzymes, antioxidants and trace mineral activators. They act as catalytic enzymes for the biochemical reactions of the body[24].

The functional components of the vitamin C complex include ascorbic acid as well as the vitamin P and K factors. As mentioned, ascorbic acid is the antioxidant or protector of the vitamin complex. As an antioxidant, it is used in the body to help combat free-radical activity as well as for the formation of certain enzymes. Vitamin P was named by Albert Szent-Gyorgyi, a Hungarian physiologist, who won the Nobel Prize in 1937 for the discovery of vitamin C. Today the vitamin P factors are known as bioflavonoids. They include citrin, hesperidin, rutin, flavones, flavonals, catechin, and quercetin. These are the antihemorrhagic or anti-scurvy portion of the C complex. Their function is to give strength to the capillaries walls and to regulate their permeability. The vitamin P factor is also needed to prepare serum calcium to promote coagulation for connective tissue formation.

Another component of the vitamin C complex is the vitamin K factor which promotes thrombin synthesis in the liver.

---

24 Richard Murray, "What is a Vitamin," (R. Murray and Associates, Inc., 1987), 1.

Tyrosinase, a copper containing enzyme, is the trace mineral activator of the vitamin C complex[25].

These functional components are all necessary for proper absorption and assimilation of vitamin C in the body. Taking a high-potency synthetic or crystalline extract of ascorbic acid can potentially cause a deficiency of these synergistic cofactors. If they are not in the diet of the patient who is ingesting ascorbic acid, the body will actually rob these cofactors from the tissue to use for the assimilation of the ascorbic acid.

Vitamins in nature have a specific rotational "spin." Synthetic vitamins are usually a racemic blend of left (levo) and right (dextro) "spinning" molecules. Remember, vitamins act as catalyst in the body for biological functions to occur. For them to be used as a catalyst in the body they must have the proper rotational spin. A wrong rotational spin would be like putting a left hand glove on the right hand. It does not fit and it will not work as a catalyst. Therefore, even when all of the cofactors are available, the best functional digestive system will only be able to utilize half the synthetic vitamins in each dose. The rest will be excreted out in the urine or feces. Hence, the advantages of using fresh whole foods and food-based supplements.

Vitamin C is found in citrus fruits, berries, cherries, tomatoes, red peppers, raw mushrooms and potatoes. The anti-scorbutic phytochemicals of the vitamin P factor (bioflavonoids) are found in red peppers, buckwheat, blueberries, the OPCs (oligomeric procyanidins) and citrus fruit (abundantly in the rinds). It is best

---

25 "Cataplex C as Compared with Synthetic Ascorbic Acid," Form VP 301(R), Vitamin Products Company, Milwaukee 3, WI.

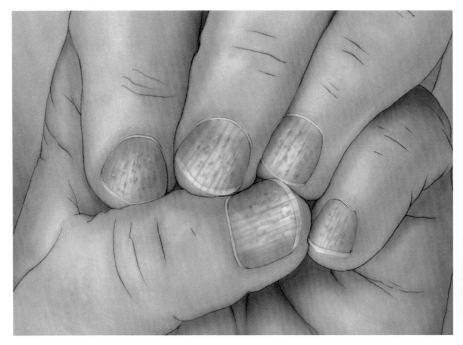

FIGURE 38. Pitting of the nails

to eat these foods fresh and raw, for the vitamin C content is diminished by oxidation and high temperatures of cooking.

Pitting

PITTING OF THE NAILS IS WHEN SMALL DENTS OR PITS OCcur on the surface of the nail plate. Pitting of the nails can be associated with alopecia, psoriasis, dermatitis or certain arthritis and connective tissue disorders[26]. The following discussion will cover them all in detail.

Pitting and Alopecia

IF THE PITTING IS ASSOCIATED WITH ALOPECIA, OR HAIR loss, it is important to determine and treat the underlying cause.

26 Robert S. Fawcett, Sean Lanford, Daniel L Stulberg, "Nail Abnormalities: Clues to System Disease," *American Family Physician* (March 15, 2004).

Some common causes of hair loss are nutritional deficiencies, under or over-active thyroid function, stress, hormonal imbalances, autoimmune diseases, chemotherapy, radiation, pharmaceutical drugs, infections of the scalp or inflammation of the hair follicles. In all cases nutritional support should be used in tandem with any other treatment.

In one month's time healthy hair will grow about a half inch. The hair follicle is made up of protein and fatty acids. The hair shaft or fiber (like the fingernails) is composed of keratin and other amino acids, fatty acids, lipids, trace minerals (especially sulfur), melanin, salt and water. These all need to be abundant in the diet for a patient to have healthy hair.

Proteins, or more specifically amino acids, are the main constituent of the hair fiber. They promote hair growth while providing strength and elasticity to the hair. The hair follicle produces keratin from amino acids available in the blood. It is important to have the patient eat a variety of protein-rich foods to ensure all the necessary amino acids are available for healthy hair production. Also make sure the patient has optimal protein digestion. Patients on acid blockers or antacids, those who have had stomach stapling or stomach bypass surgeries, patients with ulcers and other digestive ailments will have compromised protein digestion. Consider supplementing with a digestive aid high in betaine hydrochloride for these patients.

Healthy fats—lipids, cholesterol, fatty acids as well as fat-soluble vitamins—nourish the hair's root and contribute to the hair's sheen and tensile. Healthy fats include a balance of naturally saturated fats (from meat, dairy, coconut and palm kernel) along with unprocessed and cold-pressed, monounsaturated fats (primarily omega-3 fatty acids from fish, nuts and vegetable source) and unprocessed and cold-pressed, polyunsaturated fats (primarily omega-6 fatty acids from seed or vegetable source). Complement your patient's diet with a flax, fish, or wheat germ oil supplement. Belching and indigestion after eating fatty or oily foods are indications of biliary (bile) insufficiency, stasis, or blockage. Beets, beet greens and spinach contain betaine which thins the bile, enabling it to flow. Herbal cholagogues/choleretics such as dandelion root (*Taraxacum officinalis*), Oregon grape root (*Mahonia spp.*) and greater celandine (*Chelidonium majus*) may also be used. (Check for contraindications and drug interactions.) For patients with a cholecystectomy (gallbladder removed) recommend a bile supplement to be taken with meals to ensure complete digestion and assimilation of their fats and fat-soluble vitamins.

Sulfur is responsible for binding the amino acids together in the hair fibers, bestowing to the hair its durability and resistance to degradation. Foods rich in sulfur include cabbage, broccoli, kale, Brussels sprouts, cauliflower, garlic, onions, leeks, chives, shallots, turnips, radishes, and mustard greens. Eating these vegetables will also provide an array of other trace minerals and salt that is necessary for production and health of hair.

Water is essential for growth of normal and healthy hair. The water in the hair contributes to its moisture and healthy appearance. The hydrophilic amino acids in the hair fiber attract and bind water to them. Water is so necessary that the hair will actually absorb moisture from the humidity in the atmosphere. Six to eight glasses of pure spring or filtered water should be consumed daily.

Melanin gives color to the hair fiber. Melanin is produced in the hair follicle with the assistance of tyrosine, cysteine and the B vitamin complex. There are two types of melanin. Eumelanin is responsible for black and brown shades of hair. Phaeomelanin is responsible for blonde and red shades of hair.

In alopecia that is not induced by medical treatments, first look to the patient's diet, second to their thyroid and adrenal function. Hair is a non-essential tissue. During times of starvation and disease in order to survive, the body will send the nutrients it does have to feed and maintain the essential organs, cutting off the nutrient supply to non-essential tissue. Make sure your patient's daily diet contains adequate amounts of healthy protein, fats, complex carbohydrates, fiber, vitamins, minerals and water.

Malnutrition from fad and crash diets, vegetarianism, eating disorders such as anorexia and bulimia, gastrointestinal diseases that affect digestion and absorption of nutrients and anemia can cause hair loss. It will be necessary to support these patients with food-based supplements containing multiple vitamins, trace minerals, amino acids, essential fats, and a digestive aid to ensure adequate absorption and assimilation.

Alopecia is often related to thyroid disorders. To evaluate thyroid function and nutritional support for the thyroid gland, please refer to Chapter 2 under *Thick Tongue* and in this chapter under *Terry's Nails and Hyperthyroidism.* Other endocrine imbalances that affect hair loss are an excess production of cortisol by the adrenal glands (please refer to *Clubbing* associated with

Emphysema for adrenal gland support) and in men, an excess of dihydrotestosterone (DHT), a testosterone metabolite.

Pitting and Psoriasis

IF THE PITTING IS ASSOCIATED WITH PSORIASIS, HAVE THE patient keep a detailed food diary. Note which foods when eaten spurred a "flare up" in the rash, and which foods eaten kept the rash in remission. Then have the patient eliminate the offending foods from their diet. Foods and substances linked to triggering flare ups in some psoriasis patients include gluten, alcohol, colas, MSG, condiments, red meat, dairy, citrus fruits, hot and spicy foods, trans fats, cigarette smoke and food preservatives/additives.

It is common for psoriasis patients to have intolerance to the gluten in grains. Remove all flours, breads, pastas and cereals for several weeks to see if the rash improves. Add lacto-fermented foods to the patient's diet or a mycelium yeast supplement to improve digestion and assimilation of carbohydrates in the large intestines. Some of these foods and beverages include yogurt, kefir, buttermilk, sauerkraut, kim chi, kvas, and pickled vegetables.

Eating foods high in omega-3 fatty acids nourishes the skin and helps dampen the inflammation and rash. Omega-3 fatty acids and eicosapentanoic acid (EPA) are converted by the body into anti-inflammation substances called series 3 prostaglandins, leucotrienes and resolvins. Foods rich in omega-3 fatty acids include salmon, tuna, scallops, halibut, cod, shrimp, walnuts, flax seeds and flax oil, cauliflower, kale, cabbage, collard greens, Brussels sprouts, mustard greens, olives and olive oil. For many patients it is beneficial to concurrently use a flax, fish or black current seed oil supplement until the psoriasis goes into remission.

Consuming hydrogenated and trans fats can exacerbate pso-riasis. To ensure complete digestion and assimilation of fats, oils and fat-soluble vitamins it may be necessary to adjunct the diet with a cholagogue/choleretic to stimulate production and flow of bile in a psoriasis patient. Some cholagogue and choleretic includ-ed herbs such as dandelion (*Taraxacum officinalis*), greater celan-dine (*Chelidonium majus*), Oregon grape root (*Mahonia spp.*) or a betaine supplement made from beets, beet tops or spinach.

It is imperative for the patient to eat ample amounts of fresh fruits and vegetables to ensure they are consuming adequate amounts of phytochemicals, vitamins A and vitamin C to nour-ish the skin and support their immune system. Keep in mind that inflammation creates a perfect environment for infections to grow and thrive. So look for and treat any associated infections.

Zinc is also necessary for healthy skin and immune function. Foods high in zinc include oysters, calf's liver, crimini mushrooms, spinach, sesame and pumpkin seeds, shrimp, beef and lamb.

Selenium, which is found in Brazil nuts, raw crimini mush-rooms, cod, tuna, halibut, shrimp, calf's liver, eggs and bar-ley, is necessary for the production of glutathione peroxidase. Glutathione peroxidase is an enzyme that hinders the formation of certain leucotrienes which can exacerbate psoriasis.

Vitamin D has been shown to be beneficial in psoriasis due to its inflammatory mediating properties. Make sure your patient is getting adequate exposure to sunlight, enabling vitamin D pro-duction by the body. Remember the rays of the sun works with the cholesterol in the skin to produce vitamin D. Vitamin D can also be found in foods such as salmon, sardines, shrimp, cod, cod liver oil and eggs. It may be necessary to adjunct the psoriasis patient's diet with food-based supplements to ensure they are getting adequate amounts of the aforementioned nutrients.

The skin is an organ of detoxification as well as the liver, kidneys, bowel and lungs. It is important to remember this biological function of the skin when dealing with skin rashes, eruptions, dermatitis and acne. After the patient has removed their triggers, cleaned up their diet, rebuilt their intestinal flora and has been in remission for a period of time, consider doing a gentle detoxification. This removes the burdens from the liver, bowel and kidneys which are increasing the detoxification demands on the skin. Detoxifying before some initial healing has taken place can exacerbate the psoriasis outbreaks. For more in-depth information on detoxification please refer to Chapter Two, *Coated Tongue*.

Pitting, Arthritis and Connective Tissue Disorders

FOR PITTING THAT IS LINKED TO ARTHRITIS AND CONNECtive tissue disorders, again look at the diet and nutritionally support the connective tissue. Arthritis should be considered a condition brought about by an over-consumption of cooked and processed foods[27]. Seventeen different amino acids are needed to make connective tissue. It is essential for all 17 amino acids to be available at the same time, four of them in the raw form, along with vitamins A, C, E, sulfur, zinc and selenium for proper connective tissue production and repair. If the patient is deficient in any of these nutrients or not eating any raw forms of protein, connective tissue problems will develop. The addition

---

27 Francis M Pottenger, Jr., *Pottenger's Cats* (San Diego, CA: Price-Pottenger Nutritional Foundation, 1995), 59.

of unpasteurized, unhomogenized milk and raw dairy products; unroasted nuts and seeds; ceviche, sushi and sashimi; and copious amounts of raw vegetables will provide raw amino acids to the diet. Sugar cane juice, raw cream and butter contain the *Wolzen* or anti-stiffness factor.

Osteoarthritis is the degeneration of cartilage that is associated with physical trauma and the normal wear and tear of the joints that occurs with aging. From a biochemical standpoint it is the inability of the connective tissue to heal and regenerate healthy cells. In rheumatoid arthritis the synovial membranes of the connective tissue become inflamed and infected. It is the inflammation process that damages the connective tissue.

All types of arthritis benefit from dietary changes. First look for food allergies, sensitivities or intolerances and omit the offending foods from the diet. Some typical foods that exacerbate arthritic symptoms are red meats, pasteurized dairy, gluten from grain product, and vegetables in the nightshade family including tomatoes, potatoes, eggplant and peppers. Next remove from the diet all refined carbohydrates, sugars, artificial sweeteners, chemical additives, hydrogenated and trans fats. This virtually includes all foods that are packaged in a box or a can.

Replace refined carbohydrates with whole grains (if the patient can tolerate gluten); canned or frozen vegetables with raw or lightly steamed fresh vegetables; refined sugars and artificial sweeteners with raw dehydrated sugar cane juice, raw honey, blackstrap molasses or maple syrup; and altered fats with healthy fats especially those from the omega-3 family. Eating a daily serving of cold water fish high in omega-3 fatty acids will provide the necessary amount. Flaxseed oil is an excellent source of the omega-3 fatty acid alpha-linolenic acid (ALA).

The arthritic diet should consist of at least 60 percent fresh raw food. Eating vegetables from the alum, cruciferous or mustard families will provide the much needed sulfur and aid in detoxifying the congested liver that often accompanies arthritis. The addition of soups and broths made with bones is an excellent way to provide some of the necessary nutrients for connective tissue support.

Don't forget the importance of drinking six to eight glasses of natural spring or filtered water to lubricate the joints and to help flush out the toxins associated with the inflammation process. Patients report an improvement in symptoms within four weeks of making these suggested dietary changes, and complete remission in three years.

The use of nutritional and herbal supplements should focus on the support, repair and regeneration of connective tissue, reducing the inflammation as well as providing relief of pain and stiffness to the patient. Keep in mind it takes 18 months to regenerate connective tissue. Augmenting the diet with a raw, lead-free, veal bone meal product will provide all the necessary amino acids in their raw state, calcium in the hydroxyapatite form, trace minerals such as sulfur and boron, as well as important enzymes, for connective tissue regeneration. The addition of a food-based vitamin A, C and E complex will provide the vitamin support necessary for healthy connective tissue and the immune system.

Selenium would be naturally occurring in a food-based vitamin E supplement. A garlic, cruciferous vegetable, or black radish supplement provides sulfur. The addition of a fish or fish liver omega-3 fatty acid supplement balances the excess of arachidonic acids contributing to the inflammatory process. Gamma-linolenic acid (GLA) from borage, black current seed, evening primrose or hemp seed oils can also be used to correct the prostaglandin cascade. All these oils work to lubricate the joints and nourish synovial fluids. A good quality glucosamine sulfate and chondroitin sulfate supplement provides cellular support and lubrication of the cartilage. If the patient does not feel improvement in three to four weeks after being on glucosamine and chondroitin, it is not a supplement they need. The use of betaine hydrochloride/digestive enzymes may be needed until the patient's digestive system adjusts to the radical dietary changes. Check and correct the pH of arthritic patients with accompanying spurring or spondylitis. Minerals, such as calcium, precipitate out of tissue if the pH is too acid or alkaline. Using an orthophosphoric acid supplement for 8 to12 weeks works well to break up calcium deposits.

Herbs traditionally used to aid in the treatment of arthritis include willow bark, boswellia, celery seed and nettle leaf *(Urtica spp.)*. Willow bark *(Salix spp.)* contains constituents that produce a salicylic acid-like reaction in the body. Salicylic acid is the main ingredient in aspirin. Willow bark has analgesic, anti-inflammatory and anti-rheumatic properties. Boswellia *(Boswellia serrata)*, better known as frankincense, is used for its anti-inflammatory and anti-arthritic actions. Nettle leaf *(Urtica spp.)* provides a

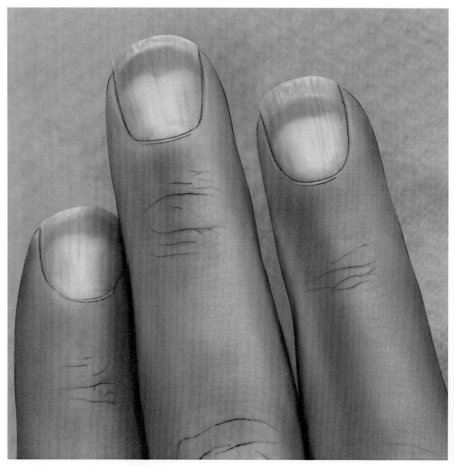

FIGURE 39. Half-and-Half nails

rich source of vitamins, minerals and anti- rheumatic properties. Celery seed (*Apium graveolens*) contains fatty acids, anti-inflammatory and anti-rheumatic constituents. Again, check any and all contraindications and drug interactions when using herbs.

Half-and-Half Nails

WITH HALF-AND-HALF NAILS, THE LUNULA, OR CRESCENT moon at the base, increase in size to encompass half of the nail plate. The other half darkens. The nail becomes half-white and half-brown. This abnormality is a very specific indication of renal failure or uremia[28].

Of course with kidney or any other organ failure, immediate medical intervention is imperative. With that being said, it is also important to provide nutritional support when the patient is able to eat or take dietary supplements. Nutrition provides the building blocks for repair and regeneration of all tissue. A supportive whole food diet and the correct nutritional supplements will assist in the healing process. A physician who checks for contraindications and interactions should not be afraid to use nutritional support with other forms of medical intervention or treatment. They truly are complimentary. Keep in mind to be judicial with your recommendations and dosing. Never burden an impaired organ or its function with nutrients.

In kidney failure and disease, dietary restrictions may be necessary. Restricting dietary proteins will reduce the accompanying nausea, vomiting and anorexia by impeding the rise of serum nitrogen levels. Foods containing potassium (bananas, potatoes, avocados, oranges, salt substitutes, etc.), phosphorus (soda, red meat, whole grains, nuts, peanut butter, etc.) and sodium (table salt, packaged and canned foods, processed meats, etc.) will need to be limited when blood or serum levels of these minerals become out of balance due to the kidneys' inability to properly process them. High blood levels of phosphorus will cause calcium to precipitate from bone and tissue. Calcium supplementation will help keep this in check.

---

28 Robert S. Fawcett, Sean Lanford, Daniel L Stulberg, "Nail Abnormalities: Clues to System Disease," *American Family Physician* (March 15, 2004).

Be sure to monitor the patient's urine pH. It is best to do this with the first void of the morning for three to five days and average out the readings. The urine pH should range between 5.5 and 6.0. Address accordingly and refer to the *Acid/Base-Producing Food Chart* in the Appendix for dietary assistance in managing the patient's pH. Metabolic acidosis accompanies kidney failure. The kidneys help to keep the acid/base balance in homeostasis by regulating the bicarbonate (HCO3) concentrations. This function fails to work properly in kidney overload. Bicarbonates are secreted in the stomach and are present in all bodily fluids. Recommend a sodium bicarbonate or potassium bicarbonate supplement in accordance with blood values. Celery root which is a rich food source of bicarbonates can be prepared and eaten as a vegetable.

Nutritional support of the kidneys should include the vitamin A and C complexes, the arginase enzyme and kidney glandulars. Vitamins A and C complexes support the epithelial and connective tissue components of the kidneys and urinary tract. Vitamin C also activates the kidney enzyme, arginase. Arginase is produced in a healthy liver and hydrolyzes arginine into urea in the kidneys to dispose of excess ammonia. Liver and kidney contain the arginase enzyme and should be added to the diet. If not eaten daily, augment the diet with a kidney glandular supplement. Peas, pea vine and its juice contain arginase precursors making them another dietary consideration.

Remember to nutritionally support the heart in kidney disease. When the kidneys are ailing, the heart acts as a back-up and helps pump all the circulating fluid in the body, increasing demand on its function.

Terry's Nails

IN CASES OF TERRY'S NAILS, INSTEAD OF THE NORMAL, CLEAR pink color, the nail plate turns an opaque white with a reddish brown distal band. The manifestation of this nail change can be associated with liver failure, cirrhosis of the liver, diabetes, hyperthyroidism, malnutrition, or congestive heart failure[29].

Terry's Nails Associated with Cirrhosis of the Liver or Hepatic Failure

IN CASES OF TERRY'S NAILS ASSOCIATED WITH HEPATIC FAILure or cirrhosis of the liver, first remove all the offending assaults. Once the patient is feeling well enough to eat, it is important to gently feed the liver. This can be done in conjunction with other medical treatment. Remember to be gentle in your approach. Never burden an ailing organ with intense nutritional therapy. The liver requires fat-soluble vitamins A, E, F and K, the G factor of the vitamin B complex, and trace minerals for regeneration of healthy tissue.

Two supplement oils that contain the necessary fat-soluble vitamins are fish liver oils and fat-soluble chlorophyll. Unfortunately, both of these oils are difficult for a patient with a deficient liver to digest and assimilate. The addition of a bile supplement or cholagogue/choleretic will be necessary to stimulate production and flow of bile, assuring proper digestion and

29 Lynn S. Bickley, Peter G. Szilagyi, *Bates' Guide to Physical Examination and History Taking* (Philadelphia, PA: Lippincott Williams & Wilkins; 2003), 110.S.

assimilation of their fatty acids and fat-soluble vitamins. Some cholagogue and choleretic include herbs such as dandelion (*Taraxacum officinalis*), greater celandine (*Chelidonium majus*), Oregon grape root (*Mahonia spp.*) or a betaine supplement made from beets, beet tops or spinach.

The vitamin G factors are found abundantly in organ meats, red meat, raw dairy and nutritional yeasts. Blackstrap molasses (2 tablespoons/day) makes an excellent trace mineral supplement. Have the patient eat liver from naturally raised calf, pig, chicken, or turkey. If they are adverse, offer a liver glandular supplement. Add to his diet foods that encourage liver detoxification— including red peppers, garlic, onions, beets, beet tops, spinach, mushrooms, radishes, asparagus, oranges, seafood, brewer's yeast, eggs and cruciferous vegetables including cabbage, broccoli, Brussels sprouts, cauliflower and kale. Please refer to the section on *White Coating*, or *hairy tongue* in the previous chapter for more information on detoxification and nutritional cleanse.

Terry's Nails and Diabetes

IF THE PATIENT WITH TERRY'S NAILS HAS DIABETES, REVIEW his diet and recommend changing to a strict whole food diet. Have the patient remove all the artificial sweeteners, refined sugars and carbohydrates and adulterated fats from their diet. This includes all chemicals and preservatives; boxed, canned, packaged and fast foods. Replace refined carbohydrates with a limited amount of whole grains and complex carbohydrates; replace hydrogenated and trans fat with cold-pressed vegetable, coconut, seed oils or butter; replace boxed, canned or package foods with fresh, raw or lightly-cooked vegetables; and replace pasteurized dairy with raw dairy products. Processed meats should be replaced with natural, pasture-raised meat/poultry and fresh water or ocean-caught fish, raw nuts and seeds. The diabetic patient will have to learn to limit their intake of all sweeteners whether they are refined, artificial or natural. A limited amount of low-glycemic, fresh, ripe fruit can be eaten to satiate sweet cravings. Consuming adequate amounts of fiber is essential for the diabetic patient. No sodas or fruit drinks, especially diet drinks with synthetic sugar substitutes, should be consumed. These will cause an increase of blood sugar levels as well. Stevia (*Stevia rebaudiana*) is an herb that does not affect blood sugar levels, making it a better alternative sweetener. A little 100 percent fruit juice mixed with seltzer or carbonated water is a satiating substitute to commercial carbonated beverages.

Doctors have reported patients with non insulin-dependent and insulin-dependent diabetes completely recovering from the condition by solely making dietary changes. Some patients have accomplished this by a low-carbohydrate, high-protein, Atkins type diet; others by a 50 percent or greater raw food, vegetarian diet. The common denominator in both these diets is the elimination of devitalized, processed foods and the addition of whole, fresh, nutritionally dense foods. Patients who make dietary changes and/or take nutritional supplements need to check their blood sugar levels daily and adjust their insulin accordingly.

Due to the over-consumption of refined, devitalized, processed foods, the diabetic patient tends to be nutritionally deficient in the very vitamins and minerals necessary to produce insulin, metabolize glucose and control blood sugar levels. These include the vitamin A, B, C, D and E complexes, chromium, zinc, magnesium, manganese, potassium, selenium and vanadium.

Vitamin A enhances delivery of insulin to the muscle tissue and improves insulin sensitivity. The vitamin B complex assists in glucose metabolism, stimulates secretion of insulin from the beta cells of the islet of Langerhans in the pancreas and improves insulin sensitivity within the cells. The vitamin C complex helps with insulin regulation by inhibiting insulin release by the pancreas. Vitamin D also plays a role in proper insulin secretion. Vitamin E protects the beta cells and enhances cell membrane permeability of insulin, increasing cellular glucose levels[30].

Chromium is part of the glucose tolerant factor which is essential for glucose metabolism and regulation. It helps in mediating the effects of insulin and enhances uptake of glucose into the cells. Zinc and magnesium are involved in insulin production, secretion and utilization. They also help maintain and protect the beta cells from destruction. Manganese improves glucose transportation and increases insulin-stimulated glucose oxidation. It is a cofactor for enzymes involved in glucose metabolism. Potassium enhances insulin secretions, response and sensitivity. Selenium works synergistically with vitamin E to protect the pancreas from damage and degeneration. Vanadium functions to

---

30 Judith DeCava, "Developing Diabetes", *Nutrition News and Views*: Vol. 4, No.3 (May/June 2000).

lower blood sugar by assisting in glucose output, transportation and breakdown[31]; [32]; [33].

Remember to check for parasites in all cases of diabetes. The pancreas recognizes the intestinal parasites as undigested protein. The presence of parasites in the intestines triggers the continual release of proteolytic enzymes from the pancreas in order to digest the protein-based exoskeleton of the parasites. This perpetual burden exhausts all functions of the pancreas including healthy insulin production and release. For more information on the eradication of parasites please refer to *Dark Circles* in Chapter One.

Pancreatic glandulars, a food-based multiple vitamin/mineral supplement, chromium with the glucose tolerance factor, and digestive enzymes will adjunctively support the diabetic patient. It is necessary to monitor blood sugar levels daily and adjust the patient's medications when making dietary changes and using nutritional supplements.

Terry's Nails and Hyperthyroidism

TERRY'S NAILS MAY ALSO BE RELATED TO HYPERTHYROIDISM. In hyperthyroidism the thyroid is producing and releasing an excessive amount of thyroid hormones. This speeds up the body's metabolic and oxidative processes. As a rule, the hyperthyroid patient tends to be thin, with a rapid pulse rate and elevated body temperature.

---

31 Ibid.
32 Michael Murray, and Joseph Pizzorno, *Encyclopedia of Natural Medicine* (Rocklin, CA: Prima Publishing, 1991), 269-295.
33 Tom Brody, *Nutritional Biochemistry* (San Diego, CA: Academic Press, 1999), 840-841.

Signs and symptoms of hyperthyroidism include:
- Weight loss
- Protruding eyes
- Dilated pupils
- Dry eyes
- Goiter
- Thyroid nodules
- Arrhythmia, tachycardia, palpitations
- Anxiety
- Irritability
- Increased perspiration
- Thin, moist skin
- Tremors
- Rapid swallowing and breathing
- Panic disorder
- Insomnia
- Muscle weakness
- Diarrhea or frequent bowel movements
  Amenorrhea
- Reduced resistance to infection
- Osteoporosis
- Certain eye conditions are also associated with hyper-thyroidism. They include:
- Edematous eyelids
- Diminished vision
- Burning and/or gritty sensation
- Proptosis
- Inability to completely close the eyelids, particularly during sleep
- Diplopia
- Reduction of color vividness

- **Inflammation and reddening of the conjunctiva**

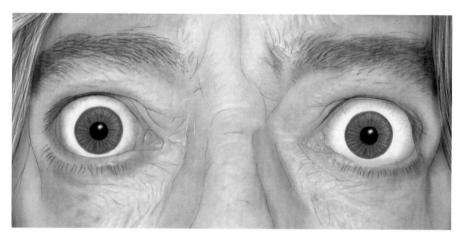

FIGURE 41. Bulging eyes of hyperthyroidism

In proptosis or exophthalmus, there is accumulation of fluid, fats and inflammatory cells causing swelling behind the eye which push the eye balls outward. This is easily distinguished from a patient with large, round eyeballs. In proptosis, you can see the whites of the eye above and/or below the iris. It is usually bilateral in hyperthyroidism.

Many thyroid conditions, whether hypo or hyper, respond well to nutritional support. The thyroid needs: vitamins A, B, C, D, E and F complexes (essential fatty acids); the amino acid ty-rosine; and the trace minerals iodine, iron, selenium, magnesium and zinc to produce and utilize its hormones. Fats transport and liberate iodine for utilization in the body. This is especially true of unsaturated fatty acids which readily combine with iodine[34].

34 F. E. Chidester, *Nutrition and Glands in Relation to Cancer* (Milwaukee, WI: Lee Foundation for Nutritional Research, 1944), 100.

Thus it is essential to consume healthy fats while supplementing with iodine.

For hyperthyroidism, it is necessary to supplement the patient as in hypothyroidism with the addition of several other nutrients. The whole vitamin C complex protects the body's proteins from the rapid oxidation rate which causes the breaking down of muscle leading to weight loss in the hyperthyroid patient[35]. Another important adjunct is yakitron. Yakitron is a liver extract, brought to our attention by the Japanese in the 1920s. This potent extract, which is a liver detoxifier and natural anti-histamine, also detoxifies the blood of excess thyroid hormones[36].

Additional information and more in-depth nutritional support of the thyroid gland can be found in the Thick Tongue, *Hypothyroidism* section, in Chapter Two.

Terry's Nails and Malnutrition

MALNUTRITION ASSOCIATED WITH TERRY'S NAILS CAN BE caused by:

- **Lack of food in the diet**
- **A diet of devitalized, processed foods**
- **Insufficient hydrochloric acid and digestive enzyme production**
- **Gastrointestinal diseases**
- **Alcoholism**
- **Anorexia**
- **Bulimia**

Check for and address any of the causation factors. The

---

35 "Vitamin C Complex," *Index of Product Bulletins* (Milwaukee,WI: Vitamin Product Company, circa 1940's).
36 "Anti-Pyrexin/Antronex," *Index of Product Bulletins* (Milwaukee,WI: Vitamin Product Company, circa 1940's).

addition of a food-based, multiple vitamin/mineral supplement as well as a digestive aid helps the patient in the interim.

Terry's Nails and Congestive Heart Failure

FOR THE PATIENT WHO HAS CONGESTIVE HEART FAILURE IN connection with Terry's Nails recommend a Mediterranean or South Beach type diet. Both of these diets nurture the heart muscle and function, eliminate the offending foods and are easy to implement.

Congestive heart failure is frequently referred to as *beriberi of the heart*. Beriberi is believed to be the Sinhalese (a dialect of Sri Lanka) word for *I can't, I can't*. It is a vitamin B1 or thiamine deficiency causing lethargy and extreme fatigue. The cardiovascular symptoms of beriberi include an enlarged heart, rapid heartbeat, fluids in the lungs and edema in the extremities. Supplemental support should include the vitamin B complex to innervate the nerves of the heart. This innervation will act to help shrink the enlarged and flaccid heart muscle enabling the valves of the heart to close properly. The vitamin G complex is necessary for its vasodilatation and lipotrophic properties which will assist in the reduction of fat and cholesterol deposits contributing to high blood pressure.

The use of a potassium, calcium and magnesium supplement will also help lower blood pressure and provide important minerals necessary for heart muscle relaxation and regulation of the heart beat by nourishing the parasympathic nervous system. The addition of heart glandulars and omega-3 fatty acids from fish, cod liver or flaxseed oil will round out the heart health protocol.

Patients with fluid retention should be on diuretics to aid in the kidney excretion of the fluids. Diuretic herbs such as parsley (*Petroselinum crispum*), nettle (*Urtica spp.*) and dandelion (*Taraxacum officinalis*) provide, rather than deplete, potassium. Remember to check for contraindications and drug interactions.

Dry, Brittle Nails

NAILS THAT ARE DRY, BRITTLE AND CRACK EASILY CAN BE

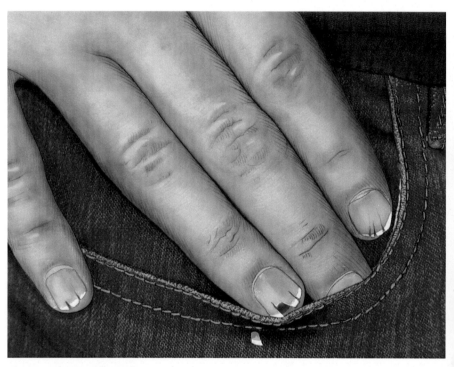

FIGURE 42. Brittle nails

correlated to a vitamin A, a vitamin F or an essential fatty acid deficiency. As stated earlier, healthy nails require protein, fats, minerals and water. The protein and minerals add strength to the nails. The fatty acids and water lubricate the nails. Look for a deficiency or assimilation problem of the latter if the patient is complaining of dry and brittle nails. Patients with a vitamin

F deficiency may have accompanying dry skin and hair. Patients with a vitamin A deficiency may remark about skin rashes, mucous membrane problems—whether it is under or over-production of mucous—and vision problems, notably night vision.

In their unadulterated form as whole foods, fat-soluble vitamins occur naturally with essential fatty acids and other lipids. Vitamins A and F occur together in foods such as raw cream, egg yolks, fish liver oils and fat-soluble chlorophyll from green plants. These foods are also high in healthy fats which are needed for lubrication of the nails.

Make sure the patient is producing and secreting adequate amounts of gastric/pancreatic lipase and bile which are necessary for proper digestion, emulsification and assimilation of fats and fat-soluble vitamins. Eating hydrogenated or trans fats will interfere with that process. Hence, eliminate all processed fats from the patient's diet. If the patient belches or gets intestinal upset after eating foods high in fats, this is an indication of a lack of lipase or biliary stasis. For these patients, recommend a digestive enzyme supplement and/or a cholagogue to aid in digestion and assimilation of fats and fat-soluble vitamins in their diet.

Also, be sure to stress to the patient the importance of drinking six to eight glasses of filtered or spring water daily to help in the hydration and lubrication of the nails. No other liquid works like pure water to lubricate and detoxify the body.

Yellow Nail Syndrome

In Yellow Nail Syndrome, the nails grow very slowly, the nail plates turn yellow, the cuticles disappear, eventually the nails become loose and can even detach as in onycholysis.

First, rule out the possibility of the nails being stained yellow from the patient smoking cigarettes. Yellow nails syndrome may accompany such conditions as impaired lymphatic drainage, lymphedema, hypoalbuminemia, sinusitis, rheumatoid arthritis, thyroiditis, tuberculosis, immunodeficiency and Raynaud's disease[37]. All of these conditions while being medically mediated can benefit long-term from proper dietary, nutritional and herbal therapies as well.

With impaired lymphatic drainage, lymphedema and other lymphatic conditions it is important to nourish the lymphatic system as well as the immune system. White blood cells such as lymphocytes and monocytes are active components of both the lymph and immune system. The lymph nodes along with macrophages (a type of monocyte found in the lymph nodes, liver and spleen) filter the lymphatic fluids. Vitamins A, B6, C and the trace minerals iodine and zinc are especially important to support the production and function of these white blood cells. Additional liver and/or spleen support may be necessary. Flaxseed oil is a light, easily digestible oil that should also be considered as a supportive in all lymphatic disorders. As an oil, it has the unique ability to thin lymphatic fluids, enabling the lymph to circulate more freely. Flaxseed oil is also an excellent systemic lubricant high in the omega-3 fatty acid alpha-linolenic acid (ALA) which is a precursor to eicosapentaenoic acid (EPA).

The use of lymphagogues and herbs which stimulate the activity of macrophages can be a useful adjunct. Lymphagogues

---

37 Robert S. Fawcett, Sean Lanford, Daniel L Stulberg, "Nail Abnormalities: Clues to System Disease," *American Family Physician* (March 15, 2004).

are herbs used to support or stimulate the lymphatic system and correlating organs. Some of these include burdock (*Artium lappa*), calendula (*Calendula officinalis*), cleavers (*Gallium aparine*), mullien (*Verbascum thapsus*) and red clover (*Trifolium pratense*). Herbal support for macrophage activity includes goldenseal (*Hydrasis canadensis*), echinacea (*Echinacea angustifolia*) and Korean ginseng (*Panax ginseng*)[38]. Again check for any contraindications and drug interactions when using herbal therapies.

Other natural therapies to increase blood and lymphatic circulation include exercise, massage, diaphramic breathing and elevation of the extremities.

Yellow Nail Syndrome and Raynaud's Disease

IF YELLOW NAIL SYNDROME IS RELATED TO RAYNAUD'S DISease, the nutritional and herbal support should be focused on enhancing blood circulation and body temperature maintenance. It is the same support used to increase blood circulation for lack of lunulas and is worth repeating here.

The use of uncoded ribonucleic acid (RNA) is a safe nutrient that thins the blood without damaging the blood vessel or the gastric mucosal lining. RNA is a template to make proteins for the repair and regeneration of tissue. Amino acids bind to RNA in the blood. The energy thrown off by that biochemical reaction heats, hence thins the blood, increasing the circulation. It is also touted as an anti-aging nutrient. RNA is found abundantly in fish especially sardines, as well as organ meats, chlorella and

---

38 Michael Murray, and Joseph Pizzorno, *Encyclopedia of Natural Medicine* (Rocklin, CA: Prima Publishing, 1991), 59.

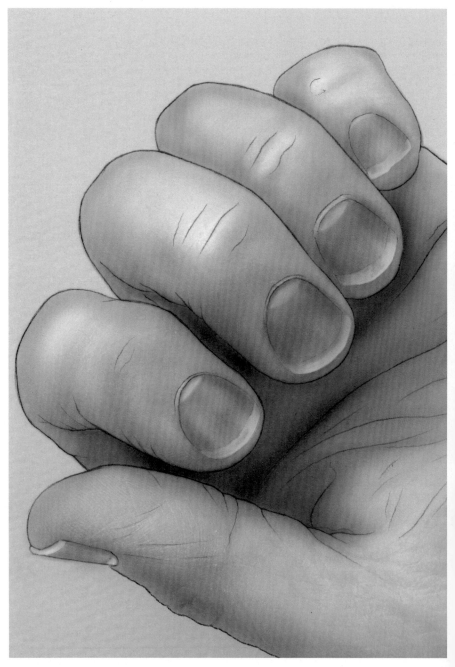

FIGURE 43. Yellow nail syndrome

nutritional yeasts. Uncoded ribonucleic acid is also available in a supplement form.

Phosphorous will improve circulation by lowering blood viscosity. Phosphorous binds with calcium in the blood to form calcium phosphate. Calcium phosphate is readily transferred from the blood into the bone. The reduction of calcium will lower blood viscosity, thinning the blood. Phosphorous will also reduce calcium deposits and plaqueing in the blood vessels and muscles, and on the bones and teeth. Phosphorous nourishes and stimulates the sympathetic nervous system. It will also increase heart rate.

Orthophosphoric acid is also available as a food supplement. When therapeutically using phosphoric acid long term, it is best to recommend a calcium supplement (taken at a different time of day than the phosphorus) to alleviate an imbalance in the calcium to phosphorus blood ratio. The use of a phosphoric acid supplement is contraindicated with a tachycardia patient or with a patient that is on a pharmaceutical blood thinner.

Some herbs to consider for Raynaud's patients are ginkgo and cayenne pepper. Ginkgo (*Ginkgo biloba*) leaf increases peripheral circulation to the limbs and brain[39] and increases oxygenation of tissue[40]. Cayenne pepper (*Capsicum spp.*) has a warming effect on the body. It has traditionally been used to improve the circulation of blood, especially gustatory and peripheral circulation. Again,

---

39 Sharon Tilgner, *Herbal Medicine from the Heart of the Earth* (Creswell, OR: Wise Acre Press, Inc., 1999), 67.
40 S. Mills and K. Bone, *Principal and Practices of Phytotherapy* (New York: Churchill Livingstone, 2000), 404.

check for any contraindications and drug interactions before recommending herbal supplementation.

Always look for and treat a heart involvement in any circulation problem. Refer to Chapter One for nutritional support of the heart. Remember, exercise is a great way to increase oxygenation and circulation of the blood.

In yellow nail syndrome associated with thyroiditis, the nails may have a more brownish tint to them. Please refer to Thick Tongue, *Hypothyroidism* section, in Chapter Two, for information on nutritional support for the thyroid gland.

For yellow nail syndrome in cases of rheumatoid arthritis (RA), please refer to the nutritional support for RA in the *Pitting of the Nails* section discussed earlier in this chapter.

Onycholysis/Plummer's Nails

ONYCHOLYSIS, OR MORE COMMONLY KNOWN AS PLUMMER'S Nails, is a term used to describe loose nail plates. The nails start separating from the distal end (or tips) of the nail bed. This painless condition may affect several or all the nails. With that said, the patient does need to be extra careful not to cause physical trauma which may lift the nail from the bed causing complete detachment which will hurt.

Onycholysis can be associated with psoriasis, physical trauma, connective tissue disorders or hyperthyroidism[41]. For information on psoriasis and connective tissue disorders please refer to these conditions in *Pitting of the Nails* discussed earlier in this chapter. Hyperthyroidism was discussed under *Yellow Nail Syndrome.*

---

41 Robert S. Fawcett, Sean Lanford, Daniel L Stulberg, "Nail Abnormalities: Clues to System Disease," *American Family Physician* (March 15, 2004).

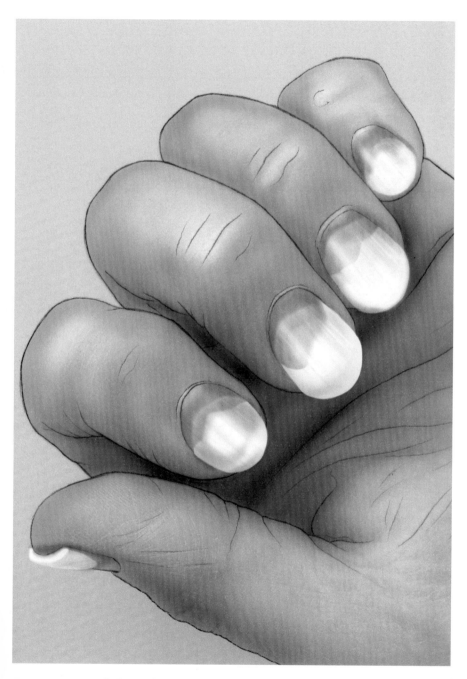

FIGURE 44. Onycholysis/Plummer's nails

Beau's Lines

WITH BEAU'S LINES THERE ARE DEPRESSIONS THAT TRANS-
verse the nail plate. They actually look like crosswise bumps and
dips in the nails. Beau's lines are usually associated with:
- **Physical trauma**
- **Parasitic infections**
- **Malnutrition**
- **Vitamin A and C deficiencies**
- **Zinc deficiency**
- **Iron deficiency**
- **Raynaud's disease**
- **Severe illnesses**
- **Illnesses associated with high fevers**

Since all the afore-mentioned have been discussed previously
in this book, please refer to the following appropriate chapters:
- **For parasites, refer to the Chapter One,** *Dark Circle.*
- **For iron deficiencies, refer to Chapter One,** *Dark Circles* **and Chapter Two,** *Pale Tongue.*
- **For zinc deficiencies, refer to this chapter under** *White Spots on the Nails.*
- **For malnutrition, refer to this chapter under** *Terry's Nails.*
- **For Raynaud's disease, refer to this chapter under** *Yellow Nail Syndrome.*

In all severe illness it is important to nourish the immune
system. The nutritional and herbal support of the immune system is similar to the support of the lymphatic system which was
discussed in the section on *Yellow Nail Syndrome.* The active
infection-fighting cells include neutrophils, lymphocytes, monocytes and macrophages. These are all part of the lymphatic fluids.

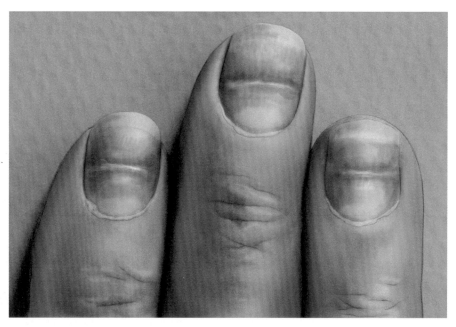

FIGURE 45. Beau's lines

Proper nutrition will support their production and function. It is recommended to add vitamin A and C complexes, calcium (especially for fevers), sulfur and thymus glandulars to the lymphatic protocol in severe illnesses.

CHAPTER FOUR

A Few Thoughts in Closing

NUTRITION IS THE FOUNDATION FOR REPAIR AND REGEN-eration of tissue and enables proper bodily functions. Eating healthfully is a wise and economical solution to the rising disease rate and the high price of health care—not only in America but worldwide.

Start to implement a whole food diet by making some simple changes. Eat a variety of fresh fruit and vegetables, whole grains, legumes, nuts and seeds, fermented foods and humanely raised meats and fish. It is imperative that the food you eat is as fresh as possible, unprocessed, unadulterated and properly prepared to maintain its nutritional value. Choose to eat fresh fruits and vegetables rather than the frozen varieties. Albeit, frozen foods maintain more of their nutritional value than canned, boxed and packaged food thus, making frozen foods a better second choice. As a rule of thumb, the more processed the less nutritional value. Organically grown is preferable over conventionally grown when it is available and affordable to buy.

To transition from a processed food diet, begin by making some simple substitutions. Replace white rice with brown (or colored) rice. Eat whole grain breads, cereals and crackers instead of white and processed. Snack on a handful of raw nuts rather than of a can of roasted and salted nuts. Substitute refined sugars with natural sweeteners. Add broth based soups to your meals several times per week, as well as wholesome yogurt and lacto-fermented foods.

Keep healthy snacks in eye sight. Place a bowl of fruit on the table. Store snacks such as pretzels, nuts, and whole grain crackers in clear glass jars on countertops or in the pantry. If good food is available over junk food, you will choose the healthier options, eventually preferring them.

It may take some time to appreciate the different tastes and textures of a whole food diet. It is important to chew your food completely before swallowing to enhance proper digestion and assimilation of the nutrients.

A good home cooked meal is a healthier alternative to eating at fast foods restaurants. Take your lunch to work. It is often more nutritious and less expensive than eating out. Try making your own breads, cookies, and desserts with whole grains, fruits, nuts, seeds and natural sugars. Keep in mind that even the most famous chefs have had culinary disasters. Continue to practice your recipes until you perfect them. Go one step further and plant your own garden. You can grow your fruit and vegetables organically. All your efforts to eat well will be rewarded by the improved quality of health you will experience.

With more women in the work force, family dynamics have changed. The working mother is often too tired to shop for and cook a proper meal. Therefore, it is important to get the whole family into the kitchen to help prepare the meals. Even small children can stir and measure ingredients. Take advantage of this family time to chat about everyone's day. Leisure time spent cooking and dining together is in jeopardy of become a lost social grace. Cooking is a critical life skill that should be learned then handed down to the younger generations.

Finally, my heartfelt thanks to the following people: To my family and friends who helped and supported this endeavor; to those professionals who contributed to the illustrations, research articles and their expertise; to my colleagues and cohorts who read, corrected, edited, and reread the manuscript. Your endearing assistance enabled me to publish this book the way I envisioned. I end this book in gratitude.

Tongue Examination for Nutritional Deficiencies Chart

Observation	Indication	Nutritional Recommendation
Purplish or magenta tongue color Painful fissures and cracks at mouth angles Atrophy of taste buds	Vitamin B2 (riboflavin) deficiency and/or Indication of blood stasis	Foods rich in vitamin B2 Food-based vitamin B2 supplement
Inflamed tongue Painful tongue Swollen tongue Fissures on lips	(Pellagra) Vitamin B3 (niacinamide) deficiency Vitamin B6 (pyridoxine) deficiency Lack of B3 formation possibly due to tryptophan deficiency	Foods rich in vitamins B3, B6 and tryptophan Food-based vitamin B3, B6 (the G factors of the vitamin B complex) Food-based amino acid supplement Brewer's Yeast
Sore tongue Sores at mouth angles Atrophy of taste buds	Iron deficiency	Foods rich in iron Food-based iron supplement
Pale or white tongue	Anemia	Foods rich in iron and chlorophyll Food-based iron supplement
	Poor circulation	See specific nutritional and herbal support for circulation
Inflamed tongue Red tongue Glossy tongue Sore tongue	Vitamin B12 (cyanocobalamin) deficiency	Foods rich in vitamin B12 Food-based vitamin B12 supplement with the intrinsic factor
"Beefy" tongue	Chi deficiency	Astragalus herbal combination formula

Tongue Examination for Nutritional Deficiencies Chart (continued)

Observation	Indication	Nutritional Recommendation
Thick tongue	Hypothyroidism and/or	Thyroid glandular supplement Kelp or iodine supplement Foods rich in array of fatty acids, Vitamin F or full spectrum FA supplement
	Pituitary deficiency in adults	Pituitary glandular supplement Foods rich in vitamin E and manganese Food-based vitamin E and manganese supplement
Geographic tongue Patchy coating Thrush	Yeast infection	Yogurt and lactic acid fermented foods Acidophilus or mycelium yeast supplement
White, coated tongue "Hairy" tongue	Sluggish digestion "Cleansing of the heat"	Cooling detoxification cleanse for 3 weeks
Atrophic Glossitis Smooth tongue with loss of papillae, Sore tongue, often	B vitamin deficiency: Riboflavin Niacinamide Pyridoxine Folate Vitamin B12 or Iron deficiency	Foods rich in all vitamin B complexes Food-based vitamin B supplement rich in the G factors Foods rich in folate and vitamin B12 Folate and vitamin B12 supplement Foods rich in iron Food-based iron supplement

Tongue Examination for Nutritional Deficiencies Chart (continued)

Observation	Indication	Nutritional Recommendation
Thick, yellow coating on tongue	Digestive problems	Tripe and stomach glandulars Foods rich in digestive enzymes Apple cider vinegar Bitters Digestive enzyme supplement Betaine hydrochloride supplement
	Constipation	Foods rich in fiber Psyllium seeds Lacto fermented foods Herbal laxatives, choleretic or cholagogue Food-based magnesium supplement
Inability to stick out tongue Short tongue Trembling tongue	Stroke or cardiac history or risk	See specific nutritional support protocols for the vascular system and heart
Gingivitis	Vitamin C complex deficiency Pre scurvy	Food rich in vitamin C and P complexes (bioflavonoids and flavanoids) Whole food vitamin C complex supplement Whole food bioflavonoid supplement, OPCs

Finger Nail Abnormalities

Observation	Indication	Nutritional Recommendation
White Spots (Leukonychia)	Zinc deficiency or	Foods rich in zinc Food-based zinc supplement
	Excessive sugar consumption	Diet low in refined sugars
Longitudinal Ridges	Vitamin F deficiency	Foods rich in a balance of the fatty acids AA, ALA, GLA, LA Food-based vitamin F supplement
Clubbing	Pulmonary or heart disease causing a depletion of oxygen in the blood	Nutritional support for the heart Nutritional support for the lungs
	Liver disease	Nutritional support for the liver
	Celiac disease	Nutritional support for the intestines
	Inflammatory bowel	Nutritional support for the bowels
Spoon Nails (Koilonychia)	Iron deficiency anemia	Foods rich in iron Food-based iron supplement Fat-soluble chlorophyll supplement
	Hemochromatosis	Support protocol for hemochromatosis
Ingrown Nails (Onychocryptosis)	Localized infection (Check for poor fitting shoes)	Apply a chlorophyll ointment or salve to affected area. Cover with a band aid. Repeat every few days until healed.
Nail Fungus (Onychomycosis)	Systemic and topical yeast infection	Mycelium yeast supplement Lacto-fermented foods Yogurt Topical daily application of white iodine or tea tree oil

Finger Nail Abnormalities (continued)

Observation	Indication	Nutritional Recommendation
Lack of Lunula	Low cellular O2 levels	Food-based iron supplement and whole vitamin E complex rich in E2 factors for oxygenation of blood and tissue
	Poor circulation	Nutrition to improve circulation
	Over use of antioxidant supplementation	Discontinue use of antioxidant supplements
Pitting	Psoriasis Alopecia Dermatitis Connective tissue disorders	See specific nutritional support protocols
Half-and-Half Nails half brown/half white nails	Specific for renal failure or uremia	Nutritional support protocol for kidneys
Dry, Brittle Nails	Vitamin F deficiency	Foods rich in vitamin F (balance of the fatty acids AA, ALA, GLA, LA) Fat-soluble chlorophyll supplement Cod liver oil, wheat germ oil
	Vitamin A deficiency	Foods rich in vitamin A Food-based vitamin A supplement
Reduced Nail Growth	Manganese deficiency	Foods rich in manganese Food-based manganese supplement
	Protein deficiency	Diet high in protein
Yellow Nail Syndrome	Impaired lymphatic drainage Lymphedema	Nutritional support protocol for lymph and lymphatic drainage
	Hypoalbuminemia	Nutritional support protocol for kidneys

Finger Nail Abnormalities (continued)

Observation	Indication	Nutritional Recommendation
Beau's Lines	Raynaud's Severe illness Trauma Parasites Malnutrition Iron deficiency	See specific nutritional support protocols
Plummer's Nails (Onycholysis)	Psoriasis Trauma Hyperthyroidism	See specific nutritional support protocols
Terry's Nails (White Nails)	Hepatic failure Cirrhosis of the liver Diabetes Hyperthyroidism Malnutrition Congestive heart failure	See specific nutritional support protocols

Mineral Relationship Chart

Mineral	Depresses
Cadmium	Copper
Calcium	Magnesium, Manganese, Phosphorous, Zinc
Chromium	Iron, Vanadium, Zinc
Cobalt	Iron
Copper	Iron, Molybdenum, Phosphorous, Zinc
Iron	Copper, Phosphorous, Potassium
Magnesium	Calcium, Phosphorous
Manganese	Iron, Magnesium, Phosphorous, Potassium
Molybdenum	Copper
Phosphorous	Calcium, Iron, Magnesium, Zinc
Potassium	Iron, Manganese, Sodium
Selenium	Copper
Sodium	Potassium
Zinc	Cadmium, Copper, Iron, Phosphorous

Acid/Alkaline Ash Producing Food Guide

Food Groups	Acid Producing Foods	Alkaline Producing Foods	Neutral Foods
Fruit	cranberries, plums, prunes	apples, apricots, bananas, berries, currents, citrus fruit (grapefruit, lemons, limes, oranges, tangerines), grapes, melons, peaches, pears, persimmons, pineapple, raisins	
Vegetables		artichokes, asparagus, beans (lima, kidney white), beets and beet greens, cabbage, carrots, cauliflower, celery, cucumbers, endive, green beans, lettuce, mushrooms, olives, parsley, parsnips, peas, sweat peppers, potatoes, radishes, rhubarb, spinach, turnips, watercress	onions
Cereals and Grains	barley, biscuits, bran, bread (white, whole wheat, rye), corn, crackers, flours, muffins, oatmeal, pastries, pastas, rice, scones		
Nuts and Seeds	peanuts	almonds, chestnuts	
Dairy	cheese	whole milk	butter, buttermilk, cream, ice cream, custard

Acid/Alkaline Ash Producing Food Guide (continued)

Food Groups	Acid Producing Foods	Alkaline Producing Foods	Neutral Foods
Meat, Fish and Poultry	bacon, beef, chicken clams, crab, duck, eggs and egg yolks, fish, lamb, liver, lobster, oysters, pork, rabbit, scallops, shrimp, veal		lard
Miscellaneous			corn oil, olive oil, honey, sugar, syrups

List of Illustrations

Index

About the Author

DONNA WILD HAS STUDIED, PRACTICED AND TAUGHT holistic health to doctors and laymen for the past 30 years. She has studied nutrition extensively at Drexel University, Colorado State University and the Lee Foundation for Nutritional Research.

Ms. Wild has owned and operated her own commercial herbal greenhouse in northern Colorado. She has written, published, broadcasted and lectured extensively on natural restorative methods for human and animal health.

Presently, Ms. Wild owns and runs Unique Perspective in Loveland, Colorado. She has a private practice, works as a consultant, lecturer and author, and lovingly tends to her organic vegetable and herb gardens.